Drug Treatment in Dementia

D0537844

Drug Treatment in Dementia

Roy W. Jones

BSc (Hons) MB, FRCP, FFPM
Director and Honorary Consultant Geriatrician
The Research Institute for the Care of the Elderly
St Martin's Hospital
Bath, UK

Honorary Senior Lecturer
School of Postgraduate Medicine
University of Bath
Bath, UK

This copy of *Drug Treatment in Dementia* is given as a
service to medicine by Shire Pharmaceuticals Ltd and
Janssen-Cilag Ltd. The views expressed herein are not
necessarily those of Shire Pharmaceuticals Ltd or
Janssen-Cilag Ltd.

Blackwell
Science

© 2000 by
Blackwell Science Ltd
Editorial Offices:
Osney Mead, Oxford OX2 0EL
25 John Street, London WC1N 2BL
23 Ainslie Place, Edinburgh EH3 6AJ
350 Main Street, Malden
    MA 02148 5018, USA
54 University Street, Carlton
    Victoria 3053, Australia
10, rue Casimir Delavigne
    75006 Paris, France

Other Editorial Offices:
Blackwell Wissenschafts-Verlag GmbH
Kurfürstendamm 57
10707 Berlin, Germany

Blackwell Science KK
MG Kodenmacho Building
7–10 Kodenmacho Nihombashi
Chuo-ku, Tokyo 104, Japan

First published 2000

Set by Graphicraft Limited, Hong Kong
Printed and bound in Great Britain
at the Alden Press, Oxford and Northampton

The Blackwell Science logo is a
trade mark of Blackwell Science Ltd,
registered at the United Kingdom
Trade Marks Registry

DISTRIBUTORS

Marston Book Services Ltd
PO Box 269
Abingdon, Oxon OX14 4YN
(*Orders*: Tel: 01235 465500
        Fax: 01235 465555)

USA
    Blackwell Science, Inc.
    Commerce Place
    350 Main Street
    Malden, MA 02148 5018
    (*Orders*: Tel: 800 759 6102
            781 388 8250
        Fax: 781 388 8255)

Canada
    Login Brothers Book Company
    324 Saulteaux Crescent
    Winnipeg, Manitoba R3J 3T2
    (*Orders*: Tel: 204 837 2987)

Australia
    Blackwell Science Pty Ltd
    54 University Street
    Carlton, Victoria 3053
    (*Orders*: Tel: 3 9347 0300
        Fax: 3 9347 5001)

A catalogue record for this title
is available from the British Library

ISBN 0-632-05492-1

Library of Congress
Cataloging-in-publication Data

Jones, Roy W., FRCP.
    Drug treatment in dementia/Roy W.
Jones.
        p.   cm.
    Includes bibliographical references and
index.
    ISBN 0–632–05492–1 (alk. paper)
    1. Dementia—Chemotherapy.
2. Alzheimer's disease—Chemotherapy.
I. Title. [DNLM: 1. Dementia—drug
therapy.   2. Alzheimer Disease—drug
therapy.   3. Dementia—diagnosis.
WM 220 J78d   2000]
RC521.J66   2000
616.8′3—dc21   99–088086

For further information on
Blackwell Science, visit our website:
www.blackwell-science.com

Contents

Foreword

As recently as five years ago there would have been little place for this book. However, the advent of pharmacological treatments for Alzheimer's disease has led to an increasing recognition that many other dementias can also be helped by a positive approach to the identification of their aetiology, and the institution of appropriate therapeutic measures.

The dementias have always been treatable, at least in part, although many working in the health care professions have traditionally adopted a rather nihilistic approach to this possibility. There must be many people with dementia who, over the years, have been denied a proper assessment and the offer of both medical intervention and support to their families, because those providing for their care believed that there was no help that could be suggested. Nothing of course is further from the truth. A careful assessment will identify those with a treatable underlying cause, albeit few in number, and also indicate worthwhile treatment strategies for others. Roy Jones' book makes these points most clearly, and also emphasizes the need to consider other therapeutic issues, for instance the management of behavioural and psychological problems.

The arrival of new treatments for Alzheimer's disease has focused the minds of many on the management of dementia in general. The need for proper assessment, in order to identify patients whose mild to moderate dementia is secondary to probable Alzheimer's disease, has opened up an appreciation of the need to respond to the problems of those whose dementia has a different cause. These drugs have, therefore, had benefits beyond the modest improvement they can offer to the significant proportion of people with Alzheimer's disease for whom they can be prescribed.

This book is a timely response to the burgeoning interest stimulated in many of us by the increasing awareness of the need for appropriate diagnosis and management. The information is easy to assimilate and is logically set out. Much of the advice is of a practical nature which will be useful in day-to-day clinical situations, and this is complemented with a discussion of the wider background that will be of interest to those who wish to set their daily tasks in the context of a broader understanding of the issues. There is no better pocket-sized book that offers so much to Doctors, Nurses, and Medical Students working with people who have a dementia, and their families. This succinct volume brings together a plethora of information, much of it buried in a multitude of symposia and papers published in a considerable number of journals, which the reader would otherwise have to search.

I am pleased to commend this overview to all who wish to deliver a better quality of care to people with dementia.

G.K. Wilcock
Professor in Care of the Elderly

Introduction

Dementia is already an international problem of enormous significance and one that is set to increase in the future. Alzheimer's disease and other dementing disorders particularly affect older people. In Western Europe, the USA and Japan more than 20% of the population are over the age of 60 and the most rapidly growing section of the population is that over the age of 85. In countries such as China and India the population is ageing even more rapidly.

The financial costs and human burden exacted by the dementias is substantial – with significant costs to health and social services in all developed countries and, increasingly, elsewhere. Some 700 000 people in the UK are estimated to be suffering with dementia including about 5% of those aged over 65 but 20% of those aged over 80.

Major scientific and medical advances in the past 15 years have increased our understanding of these conditions. Knowledge of the cholinergic deficit in Alzheimer's disease has led to the application and development of the cholinesterase inhibitors. A variety of other antidementia agents are also under active development and these are changing and exciting times.

In 1993 the cholinesterase inhibitor tacrine (Cognex) was the first drug to be approved in the USA for treating the cognitive symptoms of Alzheimer's disease. It was approved and marketed in many other countries. In 1997, donepezil (Aricept) became the first drug to be approved in the UK for the treatment of Alzheimer's disease. This was followed in 1998 by rivastigmine (Exelon) and a number of other compounds such as galantamine (Reminyl) and memantine (Akatinol) are near to approval or in development. One or more cholinesterase inhibitors are now available to patients in many areas of the world including Europe, North and South America, the Near and Far East, and Australasia.

These drugs have created opportunities and dilemmas. The potential cost of the drugs coupled with the large number of sufferers have worried many health authorities, particularly since the efficacy is not always easy to demonstrate or predict for an individual patient. On the other hand, doctors using the drugs see remarkable and obvious improvements in some patients. The drugs themselves are not complicated to use nor do they generally require special monitoring. Therefore, they should be appropriate for use by family practitioners in Primary Care. However, doctors in Primary Care are not confident about making the diagnosis of Alzheimer's disease, especially in the early stages when the differentiation from normal ageing may not be easy. The differentiation of Alzheimer's disease from other types of dementia is also a concern. The drugs therefore may be best used via shared protocols between Primary and hospital-based Secondary Care.

A book reviewing the current status of drug treatments in dementia, both in practice and in research, would appear to be timely. This book will consider the role of antidementia drugs that are primarily directed towards improvements in memory and cognitive function. It will also review the drug treatment of behavioural and psychological problems, problems that are often of more concern and significance than memory difficulties to patients and their caring families and friends. Caring for and treating people with dementia will never depend solely on drug therapy and it is important that practitioners are aware of non-drug approaches. These will be mentioned at appropriate points although it is beyond the scope of this book to consider them in detail.

The first two chapters set the scene and consider the general nature of dementia and its diagnosis. Chapter 3 considers what might be treated in dementia and how we currently measure the effects of drug treatment, particularly in the context of clinical trials that are designed to meet the requirements of regulatory authorities. The methods and instruments that are used to do this are often poorly understood by non-specialists. This can hamper any attempt to place the potential of a drug in context especially when considering an individual patient in the clinic or surgery. Chapters 4 and 5 deal with drug treatment of dementia in detail whilst Chapter 6 highlights some of the other medical problems in dementia that must not be neglected.

More general treatment considerations such as when to start and stop antidementia drug therapy, the use of guidelines and treatment protocols, quality of life and ethical issues, and some pharmacoeconomic considerations, including the number needed to treat, will be dealt with in Chapters 7 and 8. Finally, Chapter 9 considers the future and the move from symptomatic therapy to disease modification.

This book has been written for doctors working within primary and secondary care such as general practitioners, old age psychiatrists, geriatricians and neurologists. Hopefully, it will also be of value to other people working regularly with patients with dementia and their families such as community psychiatric nurses and senior staff of nursing homes.

Although the tunnel that is dementia is still long, the positive news is that many lights are now appearing.

Acknowledgements

I would like to thank everyone who has helped me in the preparation of this book. Without the patience and support of many, the task would have been impossible. This is especially true of my wife Lesley, my three sons and the staff of the Research Institute for the Care of the Elderly. Very special thanks go to my secretary Arlene Evans for her unfailing support.

List of abbreviations

AD	Alzheimer's disease
ADAS-Cog/Noncog	Alzheimer's Disease Assessment Scale—Cognitive/Non-cognitive
ADCS-CGIC	AD Cooperative Study Clinical Global Impression of Change
ADENA	Alzheimer's disease treatment with ENA-713 [rivastigmine] programme
ADL	activities of daily living
AF	atrial fibrillation
AMTS	Abbreviated Mental Test Score
APP	amyloid precursor protein
BEHAVE-AD	Behavioural Pathology in Alzheimer's Disease Scale
BPSSD	behavioural and psychological signs and symptoms of dementia
CDR	Clinical Dementia Rating Scale
CGIC	Clinical Global Impression of Change
CIBIC	Clinicians' Interview-Based Impression of Change
CNS	central nervous system
COX-2	cyclooxygenase-2
CPMP	Committee for Proprietary Medicinal Products
CSF	cerebrospinal fluid
DAD	Disability Assessment for Dementia
DLB	dementia with Lewy bodies
EPS	extrapyramidal side-effects
FAST	Functional Assessment Staging
FDA	Food and Drug Administration
GABA	γ-aminobutyric acid
GDS	Global Deterioration Scale
IADL	instrumental activities of daily living
IDDD	Interview for Deterioration in Daily Living Activities in Dementia
MALT	Metrifonate Alzheimer Trial
MAO-B	monoamine oxidase B
MMSE	Mini Mental State Examination
NGF	nerve growth factor
NNT	number needed to treat
NPI	Neuropsychiatric Inventory

NSAID	non-steroidal anti-inflammatory drug
PD	Parkinson's disease
PDS	Progressive Deterioration Scale
QOL	quality of life
RO	reality orientation
RR	relative risk
SSRIs	selective serotonin reuptake inhibitors
VaD	vascular dementia

1 The dementia syndrome

Dementia was defined by Lishman [1] in 1978 as 'an acquired global impairment of intellect, memory, and personality but without impairment of consciousness'. In fact, dementia is now more appropriately considered as a syndrome of acquired loss of cognitive function, behavioural changes and loss of social function.

The presence of memory impairment is necessary for the formal diagnosis of dementia (e.g. DSM-IV [2]), although it may not be prominent in every case in the early stages, particularly with conditions such as dementia with Lewy bodies (DLB) and subcortical dementias (see Chapter 2). The formal diagnosis also requires that the decline in memory and other cognitive functions is sufficient to affect daily life.

In most cases, dementia is progressive and irreversible. It can potentially be reversed or arrested (e.g. by surgical treatment of normal pressure hydrocephalus) but longitudinal studies from dementia clinics suggest that only 11% of dementias resolve, 3% fully and 8% partially [3]. It is likely that the true incidence of reversible dementias in the community is even lower than this.

Terminology

The terms 'presenile' (onset before the age of 65) and 'senile' dementia, in common use in the 1960s and 1970s, are now best avoided. At that time, Alzheimer's disease (AD) was considered to be the main cause of the rare presenile dementias that occurred in middle life. Senile dementia was thought to occur as a result of cerebral atherosclerosis. Postmortem studies then demonstrated that many patients with senile dementia in fact showed the typical neuropathological changes of AD.

The current view is that AD is the commonest cause of dementia in adults no matter what their age. The rather vague and abusive term 'senile' has been replaced by a specific condition. This in turn has focused research and publicity in a positive way such that few people are now unaware of the term 'Alzheimer's disease'. Nevertheless it is important to remember that all dementia is not AD; as our knowledge progresses, there will be a continuing subdivision of the dementia syndrome into a number of specific diseases with differing aetiology, pathology, neurochemistry and treatment. The main causes of dementia are shown in Table 1.1. The neuropathology of the commoner dementias will be discussed later in this chapter while clinical features of the different conditions will be discussed in Chapter 2.

Table 1.1 The main causes of the dementia syndrome

Cortical	Alzheimer's disease
	Frontotemporal degeneration including:
	Pick's disease
	Frontotemporal dementia
	Progressive non-fluent aphasia
	Semantic dementia
	Alcohol
Subcortical	Multi-infarct (white matter) dementia
	Parkinson's disease
	Progressive supranuclear palsy
	Huntington's disease
	Normal pressure hydrocephalus
	AIDS-related dementia
Cortico-subcortical dementia	Vascular dementia
	Dementia with Lewy bodies
	Corticobasal degeneration
Generalized	Prion diseases including Creutzfeldt–Jakob disease
Other	Metabolic–toxic including:
	hypothyroidism
	vitamin B_{12} deficiency
	drugs/metals
	Infections including neurosyphilis

Epidemiology

Dementing disorders mainly affect people who are old or very old. Exact estimates of prevalence vary according to the definition, the specific threshold used and the population being assessed. For example, as many as 50% of people or more in nursing homes have some degree of dementia. Prevalence rises dramatically with age, affecting less than 0.1% of people aged 40 years, 5–8% of individuals over age 65, 15–20% of those over 75 and 25–50% of those over 85 [4]. The general view is that despite the methodological differences between studies there is a consistent relationship between prevalence and age with rates doubling every 5 years.

Prevalence studies cannot distinguish between differences in the occurrence of and survival from a disease. For this reason, community-based studies of the incidence of dementia may be preferable [5]. However, there are fewer such studies available and they have given

Table 1.2 Relative frequency of different dementias. Adapted from [6]

Cause	Onset before age 65 (%)	Onset after age 65 (%)
Alzheimer's disease	34	55
Vascular dementia	18	20
Dementia with Lewy bodies	7	20
Frontotemporal dementia	12	
Other causes	29	5

very variable results. The overall incidence rate is believed to be 1.1–1.6% in the over-65s as a whole but the figures rise steeply with age.

In the USA, dementia currently affects around 6 million people. By 2001 it is predicted that there will be 364 000 cases of dementia in Canada and more than 700 000 in the UK, two-thirds of whom will be over the age of 80. The number of elderly people is rapidly increasing in the developed and, to an even greater extent, in the developing world. Dementia and, in particular, AD are therefore destined to be major health problems in the new millennium.

AD is the commonest dementia. Increasing evidence is emerging to suggest that vascular factors may contribute to the development of clinical dementia in AD. Vascular dementia (VaD) itself is, in any case, probably the next most common dementia both in the community and in specialized clinics; the exact prevalence is unknown.

Some evidence suggests that the relative proportions attributed to AD and VaD differ between populations. In Europe and North America over 50% of cases have been attributed to AD compared with 12–30% for VaD. In Asian populations, VaD appears to be more common, affecting up to 60% of patients. These differences may be spurious, reflecting different methodology and other factors.

Other types of dementia account for the smaller remaining fraction of the total, although some studies have suggested that DLB may be as prevalent as VaD in older-onset subjects. The relative frequencies of the commonest dementias (Table 1.2) differ between the earlier-onset group and the later-onset group, although AD is the commonest diagnosis in both groups The coexistence of more than one type of dementia is not uncommon. This has long been accepted for VaD and AD within the concept of mixed dementia. There is also a significant clinical (and pathological) overlap between AD, Parkinson's disease (PD) and DLB.

Genetics

Genetic factors may either be causative for a dementia or they can increase susceptibility to it.

Causative genes are responsible for a small number of cases of AD that occur in a familial autosomal dominant way usually affecting younger adults in their 40s or 50s. There are now at least six known genetic routes to AD involving mutations on chromosome 1, 14 or 21. They all appear to alter processing of amyloid precursor protein (APP) in some way such that an increased amount of the 42(43) amino acid peptide Aβ42(43) is produced. This appears to lead to the deposition of insoluble amyloid that can then precipitate all of the other features of the disease.

In contrast, some genes do not cause AD but do increase susceptibility to the disease. Most interest has centred on the apolipoprotein E (ApoE) genotype. Three forms of ApoE exist. The ApoEε3 allele is the most common followed by ApoEε4 then ApoEε2 (there is no ApoEε1). A higher frequency of ApoEε4 has been found in AD. There is a dose effect with each copy of ε4 bringing the age of onset of the disease forward by 4–5 years. Interestingly the presence of ε2 may protect subjects from AD. The presence of an ApoEε4 allele increases the accuracy of the clinical diagnosis of AD from about 85 to 90% in people with cognitive impairment. However, it is not helpful for predicting AD in cognitively normal people and a person can have histologically confirmed AD even in the absence of ε4.

The ApoE story is of interest when considering the drug therapy of AD because there have been suggestions that ApoE status may affect an individual's response to a cholinesterase inhibitor like tacrine. This needs further investigation but would be valuable if it allowed the early identification of those most likely to respond to a particular drug.

Neuropathology and neurochemistry

Some knowledge of the neuropathology and neurochemistry of dementia, particularly AD, is helpful as a basis for understanding the rationale behind treatment approaches.

Neuropathology

Careful observation of the pathological features associated with dementia has undoubtedly advanced our clinical knowledge and in particular shown that AD is responsible for most dementia whatever the patient's age. The exact diagnosis can only be confirmed by histological examination usually at post mortem and this is rarely performed. This is unfortunate since our knowledge is still inadequate and the clinical diagnosis may well be wrong.

Cerebral atrophy and loss of neurones are common to most dementias. However, it is the distribution of pathological and biochemical disturbances that determine the clinical manifestations. Although AD is usually referred to as a global decline in cognitive function, in fact, whatever the type of dementia, neither the pathology nor the cognitive deficits are ever truly global or diffuse. The underlying pathology always has a predilection for particular areas of the brain (and neuropsychological testing may also show some localization of changes in early dementia). Clinical features will depend on how focal the lesion is (e.g. after a single large stroke) and whether the dementia affects mainly cortical areas as in AD, subcortical structures as in the dementia associated with PD or a mixture as in DLB.

In AD, cortical atrophy affects all lobes of the cerebral cortex but particularly the medial temporal lobes. Alzheimer established the pathological hallmarks of AD when describing the changes in a 55-year-old woman with dementia in 1907. Currently, the main changes are considered to be those shown in Box 1.1.

BOX 1.1 Pathological features of Alzheimer's disease
- Cerebral atrophy
- Extracellular neuritic plaques with an amyloid core
- Intracellular neurofibrillary tangles formed from deposits of a protein, tau
- Synaptic and neuronal loss especially of cholinergic neurones, particularly those in the basal nuclei and the hippocampus
- Amyloid angiopathy
- Acute-phase reactants and localized inflammatory reaction

The characteristic lesions in PD are Lewy bodies in the substantia nigra. They are spherical, intraneuronal inclusions with an outer paler halo and an inner more intensively staining eosinophilic core. In DLB, Lewy bodies are also found in the cerebral cortex where they are smaller and tend to be found in small and medium-sized pyramidal cells in the deeper cortical layers.

In some dementias the atrophy is more focal and disproportionately severe in one or more lobes. In frontotemporal dementia (FTD) the atrophy is mainly confined to the frontal and/or temporal lobes. The pathology is variable, including cases with classical Pick bodies (Pick's disease) and those with more non-specific loss of neurones and gliosis. There are a number of probably related conditions associated with a distinctive distribution of abnormalities. These include FTD itself, FTD with motor-neurone disease, semantic dementia and progressive fluent aphasia; in the latter two conditions the changes are more marked in the temporal lobes.

Several dementias are associated mainly with degeneration in subcortical nuclei particularly involving the basal ganglia, midbrain and brainstem structures. Disorders in this category include Huntington's disease, progressive supranuclear palsy, corticobasal degeneration and PD.

Vascular dementia is pathologically heterogeneous. It includes dementia due to cumulative large-vessel infarcts, cumulative small-vessel infarcts (lacunar state), and so-called Binswanger encephalopathy (where the condition is usually a consequence of hypertension). Leukoaraiosis described on neuroimaging (see Chapter 2) has a less consistent association with neuropathology.

Neurochemistry

Many neurochemical studies have been carried out in AD, particularly looking at specific neurotransmitters. Interpretation has been difficult because most studies rely on post-mortem material, usually in patients with end-stage disease and where there may be confounding factors such as drug therapy at the time of death that would not be present in control tissue.

The cholinergic hypothesis

Abnormalities have been reported in a range of neurotransmitters, although the changes in acetylcholine appear to be particularly significant and consistent. It is likely that these changes are secondary to neuronal damage and death. However, by analogy with PD, it should be possible to develop replacement therapies that can enhance residual synaptic activity. Such therapy whilst important would generally only be expected to provide symptomatic therapy.

The cholinergic hypothesis suggests that AD results from a selective loss in cholinergic neurones, particularly in the basal forebrain and neocortex. This results in decreased acetylcholine levels. The known effects of anticholinergic drugs in humans and the correlation between markers of cholinergic activity, the clinical severity of the dementia,

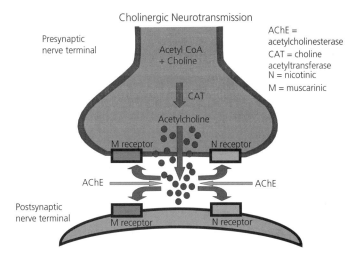

Fig. 1.1 Central cholinergic neurotransmission: key elements

and possibly some of the pathological changes in the brain provide support for the hypothesis.

Further support comes from studies in PD and DLB. In PD patients with cognitive impairment, there is cell loss in the cholinergic basal nucleus and a cortical deficit in acetylcholinesterase that is independent of any coexisting AD and correlates with the severity of dementia. Similarly, patients with DLB also show a severe loss of choline acetyl transferase in the cerebral cortex. This loss is actually more severe than that found in AD and again is correlated with the severity of dementia. The key elements of central cholinergic neurotransmission are shown in Fig. 1.1.

At the individual receptor level, it appears that presynaptic muscarinic (M2) acetylcholinergic receptors are deficient whereas cortical postsynaptic muscarinic (M1) receptors are normal. In addition, there is a reduction in nicotinic cholinergic receptors that also occur both pre- and postsynaptically. Presynaptic nicotinic receptors may be important in regulating acetylcholine release and probably the release of other neurotransmitters as well.

There is increasing interest in the potential benefits from nicotinic receptor activation. Direct stimulation of the receptors by nicotinic agonists may not be the best option because this may possibly result in desensitization of the nicotinic receptor [7]. An alternative may be to potentiate the response of nicotinic receptors to acetylcholine by modulating the response through an activator (allosteric) site on the receptor [7] (see also p. 54).

Therapies to enhance acetylcholine action therefore may show differences according to how they modulate cholinergic function as a whole and whether they show selectivity for particular elements of the muscarinic and nicotinic system.

The course of dementia

What is the prognosis of individuals who become demented? Few studies have provided information about this. Knowledge of time to institutionalization and survival time is important for resource planning. It is also important when advising patients and their caregivers.

Time to institutionalization

The median time to first institutionalization was 3.1 years from entry into the Consortium to Establish a Registry for Alzheimer's Disease (CERAD) study [8]; unmarried men had the shortest time. In a review of European collaborative data [9] using population-based samples of dementia cases, the odds of being in institutional care at study baseline was significantly higher for both prevalent and incident cases of dementia than non-cases. Estimates were also made for the rate of admission to institutional care at 2 and 3 years from baseline for prevalent cases and 4 years for incident cases. In general, prevalent cases of dementia had at least twice the entry rates to institutional care compared with non-cases, and subjects who became demented also had much higher rates of entry into care.

Survival with dementia

The onset of a dementing illness and its subsequent course will depend on the underlying disease process. It will also depend on the severity at the time of diagnosis or entry into any particular longitudinal study. Various criteria have been developed to assess severity (usually into mild, moderate or severe disease) but there is no international agreement and there is here a lack of consistency across studies. For non-institutionalized patients in Canada and the UK it is estimated that 44–49% have mild dementia, 38–46% moderate dementia and 9–13% severe dementia [10].

Two-year survival rates ranging from 37 to 86% have been reported in community studies [11] and it may be that differing diagnostic criteria explain some of the variation seen. Information from the European collaborative research study [9] showed that people with dementia (cases) had a lower survival rate than non-cases and this was consistent over time in all age groups. Women with dementia had a higher survival than men with dementia mirroring the difference in non-demented subjects. For example, 2-year survival in people aged 85 years or over was 52% for males with dementia and 76% for non-demented men whilst the equivalent figures for females were 60% and 81%, respectively. Other studies have suggested mortality rates in AD that are about three to five times more than in subjects of the same age and sex without dementia. Factors that are associated with reduced survival include being male, the presence of psychotic features such as hallucinations, and patients with physical illnesses.

In AD, progression is gradual but steadily downwards (although plateaus may occur) with an average duration from onset of symptoms to death of 8–10 years [4]. Over the years, many studies have assessed differential survival in dementia. Most have compared AD and VaD and generally show either no difference or a poorer prognosis for VaD probably reflecting the underlying vascular disease. Patients with DLB also probably have a shorter survival time than those with AD. There is few data to allow reliable comparison with other types of dementia.

Cause of death in dementia

Certification of the cause of death is notoriously inaccurate and this is particularly so with the documentation of dementia [12]. For example dementia was not mentioned on the death certificate in 30–40% of cases where dementia was known to be present in life. Although AD was the fourth or fifth most common cause of death in the USA, the US vital statistics tables did not list this or any similar term as an option.

The commonest cause appears to be related to the respiratory system, usually due to bronchopneumonia. However, patients with dementia probably die of non-specific causes, perhaps secondary to physical immobility and inanition. An increased rate of autopsy in patients with dementia would help to clarify this in addition to confirming the nature of the dementia itself.

References

1 Lishman WA. *Organic Psychiatry*. Oxford: Blackwell Scientific Publications, 1978.
2 American Psychiatric Association. *Diagnostic and Statistical Manual of Mental Disorders (DSM-IV)*, 4th edn. Washington DC: APA, 1994.
3 Clarfield AM. The reversible dementias: do they reverse? *Ann Intern Med* 1988; 109: 476–86.

4 American Psychiatric Association. Practice guideline for the treatment of patients with Alzheimer's disease and other dementias of late life. *Am J Psychiatry* 1997; 154 (5 Suppl.): 1–39.

5 van Duijn CM. Epidemiology of the dementias: recent developments and new approaches. *J Neurol Neurosurg Psychiatry* 1996; 60: 478–88.

6 Galton CJ, Hodges JR. The spectrum of dementia and its treatment. *J R Coll Physicians Lond* 1999; 33: 234–9.

7 Maelicke A, Albuquerque EX. New approach to drug therapy in Alzheimer's disease. *Drug Disc Today* 1996; 1(2): 53–9.

8 Heyman A, Peterson B, Fillenbaum G, Pieper C. Predictors of time to institutionalization of patients with Alzheimer's disease: the CERAD experience, Part XVII. *Neurology* 1997; 48: 1304–9.

9 Jagger C, Andersen K, Breteler MMB *et al.* Prognosis with dementia: results from a European collaborative analysis of population-based studies. In: Iqbal K, Swaab DF, Winblad B, Wisniewski HM, eds. *Alzheimer's Disease and Related Disorders.* Chichester: Wiley, 1999: 39–44.

10 Bosanquet N, May J, Johnson N. *Alzheimer's Disease in the United Kingdom: Burden of Disease and Future Care,* Health Policy Review Paper Number 12. London: Health Policy Unit, Imperial College School of Medicine, 1998.

11 van Dijk PTM, Dippel DWJ, Habbema JDF. Survival of patients with dementia. *J Am Geriatr Soc* 1991; 39: 603–10.

12 Burns A. Cause of death in dementia. *Int J Geriatr Psychiatry* 1992; 7: 461–4.

2 Making the diagnosis

Dementia can commence acutely, for example after a stroke. The onset can be subacute as in prion diseases such as Creutzfeldt–Jakob disease (CJD). More typically, dementia presents as a chronic, gradually progressive condition as is seen with Alzheimer's disease (AD).

In the early stages of any dementing process, the changes may be subtle and diagnosis is therefore often delayed until the disease is moderately advanced. A good history from the patient and, even more importantly, an informant who knows them well is vital.

Symptoms of dementia

The presence of dementia may be indicated by the following symptoms.
- Memory loss, predominantly for recent events.
- Difficulties with learning and retaining new information, for example forgetting recent conversations or appointments, being more repetitive and misplacing objects. In more severe dementia, people also forget previously learned material, including the names of loved ones.
- Difficulty handling complex tasks, for example cooking a meal, shopping alone or dealing with finances.
- Impairment of reasoning ability, for example dealing with abstract concepts or having a regard for the rules of social conduct.
- Impairment of spatial and visuo-perceptual ability, for example driving or getting lost in familiar places.
- Language deficits, for example difficulty finding the right words or with following conversations.
- Changes in behaviour, for example appearing more passive, being more irritable than usual or being more suspicious.

Testing for cognitive impairment

Detecting cognitive and memory impairment is easier if a standard screening instrument is used. These are described in more detail in Chapter 3 (see pp. 23–7). Even non-specialists should make themselves familiar with at least one of these. The simplest is the Abbreviated Mental Test Score but the Mini Mental State Examination is better. Asking the patient to draw a clock-face and set the hands at a particular time is a useful addition. Even if the test results are normal, they can provide a useful baseline for the future so that any decline can be documented.

Table 2.1 Diagnostic criteria for dementia (based on DSM-IV criteria)

1 Memory impairment (inability to learn new information and to recall previously learned information)
2 At least one of:
  • aphasia
  • apraxia (problems with motor activities despite intact motor function)
  • agnosia (problems recognizing or identifying objects despite intact sensory function)
  • disturbance in executive functioning (planning, organizing, sequencing, abstracting)
3 The deficits in 1 and 2 significantly impair social or occupational functioning and are a significant decline from before
4 The deficits do not occur exclusively during delirium
5 The deficits are not better accounted for by another disorder (e.g. depression, schizophrenia)

BOX 2.1 Differential diagnosis of cognitive impairment and dementia
• Delirium
• Mental retardation
• Focal impairments, e.g. amnestic disorders like Korsakoff's psychosis; aphasias
• Depression (pseudodementia)
• Drugs
• Age-related cognitive decline
• Mild cognitive impairment
• Dementing syndrome

The differential diagnosis of dementia

The first step on detecting cognitive impairment is to decide whether the patient has an underlying dementia or not. The essential features for a formal diagnosis of dementia adapted from DSM-IV [1] are shown in Table 2.1.

Delirium (acute confusion) is cognitive impairment, usually of rapid onset, associated with an alteration of attention and consciousness (see Box 2.1). Dementia must also be differentiated from mental retardation and specific cognitive impairments. Mental retardation represents life-long impairment. Specific focal impairments include amnestic disorders such as Korsakoff's psychosis in which memory is impaired out of proportion to any other cognitive deficits, and aphasia, a disorder of language comprehension and expression.

Depression is common in older people including those with dementia and can occasionally cause sufficient cognitive impairment on its own to suggest a dementia (so-called pseudodementia). The treatment of depression and its relationship with dementia is discussed in more detail in Chapter 5 (p. 81). Many drugs can either mimic or complicate a dementing process by causing confusion and cognitive impairment. Drugs with anticholinergic properties are most often responsible (see Chapter 6, pp. 92–3).

There is increasing interest in milder memory and cognitive changes that are commonly reported by many older people. People complaining about their memory and who have minor changes on formal testing may have age-related cognitive decline (ARCD). Those with slightly more abnormalities on formal testing but who still do not qualify as having a dementia are said to have mild cognitive impairment (MCI). It appears that about 15% per year of the latter group go on to develop dementia. Patients with ARCD and MCI can be classified using severity scales such as the Clinical Dementia Rating Scale or the Global Deterioration Scale, which are described in Chapter 3 (p. 30). At present these labels are probably only of use to specialists. However, studies are in progress to see whether anticholinesterase inhibitors can delay the progression of MCI to dementia; if they do, then the identification of ARCD and MCI will become more important.

In the early stages of a dementing process, differentiation from some of the processes described above may be difficult. Following the patient over a period of time may be the only way to clarify the situation. A detailed review of this area is beyond the scope of the present book.

The causes of dementia

There are more than 50 causes of a dementia syndrome, many of which are rare. The main causes have already been listed in Table 1.1 (see p. 2). AD accounts for 50–60% of dementias, with vascular dementia (VaD) and dementia with Lewy bodies (DLB) responsible for most of the remainder. Considerable overlap can occur where features of more than one condition are found producing a mixed dementia syndrome. Other important dementias to consider are frontotemporal dementia (FTD) and subcortical dementia. Prion dementias such as CJD are important but currently the number of cases is small.

AD is by far the most significant condition and the drug treatment that has been developed for dementia so far has primarily been directed towards this (see Chapter 4). Some information is presented about the other main causes both to put AD into context and because their treatment will also be considered briefly in Chapter 4.

Alzheimer's disease

Using DSM-IV criteria, the diagnosis of AD is made by identifying the features listed in Table 2.1 (see p. 12) together with two additional features. Firstly, the onset of the problems should be gradual with continuing decline. Secondly, the cognitive deficits should not be explained by other causes of dementia. This implies that AD is a diagnosis that is made after everything else has been excluded. In clinical practice, AD is usually considered as the most likely cause based on the clinical history, and this is confirmed after all other causes have, as far as possible, been excluded.

There are formal criteria to decide whether AD is definite, probable or possible [2]. Definite AD is an uncommon diagnosis in life because it depends on histological confirmation. Probable AD can be diagnosed if the dementia has been properly documented and there are deficits in two or more areas of cognition; decline is progressive; there is no disturbance of consciousness; the onset is between the ages of 40 and 90 years; and there is no other systemic disorder that could account for the dementia. A diagnosis of probable AD is supported by a deterioration in language, motor skills and perception; impaired activities of daily living and altered behaviour; a positive family history; and cerebral atrophy on computed tomography (CT) with progression documented by serial observation. The diagnosis of possible AD is made if there are variations in the onset, the presentation or in the clinical course, and if there is a second disorder that would be sufficient to produce dementia but it is not thought to be the cause.

Non-Alzheimer's dementia

Vascular dementia

VaD [3] probably accounts for around 10–20% of dementia, although vascular factors may be relevant in many more cases than this. VaD is a rather vague term that is currently under active re-evaluation. Clinically, VaD can present in several different ways reflecting the diversity of stroke mechanisms. The generic term 'multi-infarct dementia' (MID) is better reserved for those cases where it is clear that multiple small infarcts are responsible for the problems.

VaD can be caused by single large infarcts, numerous lacunar infarcts and infarcts in strategic regions such as the thalamus. Features of vascular dementia include:

- typically sudden onset and stepwise course of cognitive decline;
- history of strokes and/or transient ischaemic attacks;
- patchy cognitive impairment;
- focal neurological deficits on examination (such as hemiparesis, sensory loss or extensor plantar response);
- a source of thromboembolism (such as carotid artery disease or atrial fibrillation);
- presence of associated atherosclerosis and/or hypertension;
- neuroimaging evidence of cerebral vascular disease.

Hypertension is probably the strongest risk factor for vascular dementia (and may also be associated with AD [4]). Patients with diabetes are also at increased risk of vascular disease and stroke disease including MID.

Problems can occur with the diagnosis especially where AD and VaD coexist. It can be difficult to establish the role of vascular lesions (such as white-matter lesions or 'leukoaraiosis') identified by neuroimaging. It also appears that VaD can present in a more slowly progressive way. Finally, a recent report [5] showed that patients with AD coincident with brain infarcts (particularly if subcortical) had poorer cognitive function than those without such lesions.

Dementia with Lewy bodies

DLB is the preferred name for this condition that has become increasingly recognized over the past few years. In hospital research series, it may be commoner than VaD, although community-based prevalence rates are still unknown. Consensus diagnostic criteria have been published [6]. The main features are dementia in association with:

- fluctuating cognition with pronounced variations in attention and alertness (memory impairment may be less marked initially);
- cortical and subcortical features neuropsychologically with cognitive slowing, impaired executive function and problem-solving, and reduced visuo-spatial abilities;
- visual hallucinations (often detailed and of people and animals);
- mild parkinsonism (but tremor is uncommon).

Other features may include:

- repeated falls;
- syncope;

• delusions;
• neuroleptic sensitivity (with an adverse and extreme reaction to neuroleptics that may affect up to 50% of cases, and inadvertently be very supportive of the diagnosis).

Frontotemporal dementia

FTD is now preferred to the older term 'Pick's disease' to identify patients with focal frontal and/or temporal lobe atrophy. It also includes frontal lobe dementia with or without motor-neurone disease and the primary aphasias. FTD is the commonest dementia after AD and VaD in subjects under the age of 65, responsible for around 10% of cases.

The core diagnostic features of FTD [7] include the following.

1 Behavioural disorder:
   • insidious onset and slow progression;
   • early loss of personal and social awareness (including poor personal hygiene and misdemeanours such as shoplifting);
   • early signs of disinhibition (e.g. sexual, violent);
   • mental rigidity and inflexibility;
   • hyperorality, stereotyped and perseverative behaviour;
   • distractability and impulsivity.
2 Affective symptoms:
   • depression, anxiety;
   • hypochondriasis;
   • emotional unconcern and inertia.
3 Speech disorder:
   • progressive reduction and stereotypy of speech;
   • echolalia and perseveration.
4 Physical signs:
   • early primitive reflexes and incontinence;
   • late akinesia, rigidity, tremor;
   • low and labile blood pressure.

Subcortical dementia syndromes

Unlike AD, which is mainly a cortical dementia, some dementias involve mainly subcortical structures such as the basal ganglia, midbrain and brainstem instead of, or as well as, the cerebral cortex. These conditions lack the features such as aphasia, apraxia and agnosia traditionally associated with cortical dysfunction. Instead the dementia is associated with a slowing of information processing, poor concentration, indecision and prominent changes in personality (typically apathy and inertia) and mood (with depression being common). Language is often normal except for dysarthria and a reduced output.

The main causes of subcortical dementia are as follows.

1 Degenerative:
   • progressive supranuclear palsy;
   • Huntington's disease;
   • Parkinson's disease;
   • corticobasal degeneration.
2 Vascular:
   • lacunar state;
   • Binswanger's disease (diffuse leukoaraiosis).
3 Metabolic:
   • Wilson's disease;
   • hypoparathyroidism.
4 Demyelination:
   • multiple sclerosis;
   • AIDS dementia complex.
5 Other:
   • normal pressure hydrocephalus.

Subcortical dementias are important to recognize because, at least in some cases, effective treatments are available.

Treatable causes of dementia

There are a number of conditions that can cause a dementia syndrome where treatment can be effective, either reversing the problem completely or partially, or at the least, preventing further decline. The main conditions are listed in Table 2.2.

Investigations

Although the diagnosis of dementia is made clinically, some investigations (Table 2.3) are necessary in all patients to ensure that a potentially treatable condition has not been missed.

Abnormal laboratory values are found quite frequently when people with suspected dementia are investigated. Unfortunately this is often only a reflection of the age of such subjects. For example, abnormalities in thyroid function and vitamin B_{12} (usually in the absence of a macrocytosis) are common. Whilst it may be important to treat such abnormalities to prevent future health problems, it is unusual to find that this results in any significant improvement in the dementing disorder.

Table 2.2 Treatable causes of dementia

Deficiency states
Vitamins B_{12}, folic acid, B_1

Endocrine disorders
Hyper-/hypothyroidism
Hyper-/hypoparathyroidism
Cushing's syndrome
Addison's disease

Infections
AIDS dementia complex
Syphilis

Toxins
Alcohol
Drugs
Heavy metals

Other
Subdural haematoma
Normal pressure hydrocephalus
Depression (pseudodementia)

Table 2.3 Basic laboratory investigations in suspected dementia

Routine	Full blood count (particularly haemoglobin and MCV)
	Plasma viscosity (or ESR)
	Vitamin B_{12} and red cell folate
	Biochemistry (urea and electrolytes, LFTs, glucose, calcium)
	Thyroid function
	Syphilis serology
	Urinalysis
Occasional	γ-glutamyl transferase
	HIV

MCV, mean cell volume; ESR, erythrocyte sedimentation rate; LFT, liver function test; HIV, human immunodeficiency virus.

Neuroimaging

A number of neuroimaging techniques are useful in dementia. They include structural imaging with CT and magnetic resonance imaging (MRI) and functional imaging with single-photon emission computed tomography (SPECT).

None is diagnostic for AD and the value of brain imaging, especially in an older person with a typical clinical history and findings, is unfortunately limited. CT or MRI will reveal tumours, strokes, haemorrhages, hydrocephalus, ischaemia and other lesions that might otherwise be missed but some clinical features would usually accompany these. Angling the scan to view the medial temporal lobe can increase the value of a CT scan in AD. Serial measurements showing a reduction in the thickness of the medial temporal lobe have been used in research studies but this is not realistic for routine clinical use at present.

A SPECT scan is still not appropriate as the first-line investigation in AD except where FTD is the major differential diagnosis; SPECT can be diagnostic in FTD with the demonstration of profound anterior cerebral hypoperfusion. Its use should be reserved for those cases where the clinical picture is unclear or where medial temporal lobe atrophy is mild.

If CT and SPECT are combined in suspected AD then diagnostic accuracy can be increased. MRI can be especially helpful where VaD or normal pressure hydrocephalus is suspected.

Although a combination of structural and functional imaging appears to allow very accurate diagnosis, it is too costly and too poorly understood for routine use at present. As specific treatments become available, more precise diagnosis may be necessary, helpful and cost-effective.

Other investigations

Electroencephalography

Electroencephalography (EEG) mainly reflects cortical electrical activity. In general, diffuse brain disease produces widespread EEG changes whereas focal disease produces more localized alterations.

The EEG is rarely diagnostic but is sometimes helpful. In AD the abnormalities may be diffuse and non-specific in the early stages but progressive slowing occurs later. In contrast, it is usually normal in FTD even when the dementia is quite severe. The EEG can be diagnostic in CJD revealing a characteristic pattern with regular sharp waves.

Lumbar puncture

It may occasionally be necessary to do a lumbar puncture to clarify the diagnosis, for example in the case of a patient with positive serological tests for syphilis. Diagnostic lumbar puncture in elderly people is not a particular problem and is done as an outpatient procedure in some countries.

Cerebrospinal fluid pressure monitoring (preferably for 24 h) is used in suspected cases of normal pressure hydrocephalus, an uncommon progressive dementing syndrome, to confirm the diagnosis.

References

1 American Psychiatric Association. *Diagnostic and Statistical Manual of Mental Disorders (DSM-IV)*, 4th edn. Washington DC: APA, 1994.
2 McKhann G, Drachman DA, Folstein M, Katzman R, Price DL, Stadlan EM. Clinical diagnosis of Alzheimer's disease—report of the NINCDS-ADRDA work group under the auspices of Department of Health and Human Services task force on Alzheimer's disease. *Neurology* 1984; 34: 939–44.
3 Amar K, Wilcock G. Vascular dementia. *BMJ* 1996; 312: 227–31.
4 Hofman A, Ott A, Breteler MMB *et al.* Atherosclerosis, apolipoprotein E, and prevalence of dementia and Alzheimer's disease in the Rotterdam Study. *Lancet* 1997; 349: 151–4.
5 Snowdon DA, Greiner LH, Mortimer JA *et al.* Brain infarction and the expression of Alzheimer's disease. *JAMA* 1997; 277: 813–17.
6 McKeith IG, Galasko D, Kosaka K *et al.* Consensus guidelines for the clinical and pathological diagnosis of dementia with Lewy bodies (DLB): report of the Consortium on DLB International Workshop. *Neurology* 1996; 47: 1113–24.
7 Brun A, Englund E, Gustafson L *et al.* Clinical and neuropathological criteria for frontotemporal dementia. *J Neurol Neurosurg Psychiatry* 1994; 57: 416–18.

3 Assessing the benefits of drug treatment in dementia

Until recently, too many people regarded dementia as untreatable. This was always too nihilistic, particularly if treatment is interpreted in the broadest sense of both pharmacological and non-pharmacological management of the patient and their immediate caregivers.

The clinical features of dementia that can be treated are not limited to memory and cognition. Patients are more likely to be institutionalized because of problems with activities of daily living or behaviour than with memory difficulties *per se*. Management of these areas can be very helpful. Finally, elderly people with dementia are still subject to medical conditions independent of the dementia. It is easy to overlook treatable conditions (e.g. urinary tract infections), assuming that all problems (e.g. incontinence) result from the dementing process.

Demonstrating treatment benefits is not easy. Legitimate goals include symptomatic cognitive or behavioural improvement as well as attempts to slow, halt, reverse or prevent the disease process. The dementia syndrome can have multiple aetiologies and pathophysiologies. It is inherently unlikely that there will be a single 'antidementia drug'. At present the available therapies appear only to act symptomatically but several approaches are being pursued that may affect the disease process. It has been suggested that some symptomatic therapies may affect the disease process but this remains unproved. Different drugs and different clinical trial designs may be needed to demonstrate disease modification.

There is still controversy as to what constitutes a useful treatment benefit and how to measure it. Is it a few points improvement on a cognitive function test or must there be an obvious change in activities of daily living or quality of life?

In a book concentrating on drug treatment, it is especially important to emphasize that drug therapy is only a part of what can be offered. However, the benefits of non-drug treatment are even more difficult to demonstrate convincingly [1].

Specific drug treatment will become increasingly important in management of the dementias. With the arrival of the first marketed drugs has come a bewildering array of assessments with complex acronyms that are not always understood, even by specialists. Yet drug treatment of dementia is destined to become an everyday matter that will usually be managed by non-specialists particularly in primary care. It will be vital to have a working understanding of the assessments used in clinical trials if clinicians are to understand published trials and the significance of information presented to them. Some assessments will also be useful in diagnosis and in the monitoring of treatment.

This chapter will consider the main assessments currently used in evaluating the potential benefit of drug treatment. The following two chapters will then consider drug therapy for the treatment of intellectual function (Chapter 4) and the management of behavioural and psychological factors (Chapter 5).

Regulatory considerations

Current regulatory guidelines usually only apply to registration of symptomatic drugs to improve cognitive function for Alzheimer's disease (AD). They do not cover vascular dementia (VaD) or other dementias, or drugs specifically for the treatment of behavioural problems associated with dementias. Guidelines have been produced by the Committee for Proprietary Medicinal Products (CPMP) [2], part of the European Community system for evaluating new medicinal products, and by the US Food and Drug Administration (FDA) [3].

The CPMP [2] recommend that the main goals of AD treatment are:
• symptomatic improvement, manifest in enhanced cognition, more autonomy and/or improvement in behavioural dysfunction;
• slowing or arrest of symptom progression;
• primary prevention of disease by intervention in key pathogenic mechanisms at a presymptomatic stage.

The guidelines then concentrate exclusively on assessment of symptomatic improvement (because 'experience is lacking, either in slowing, arresting symptom progression or in primary prevention of disease').

Improvement should be assessed in the following domains:
• cognition, as measured by objective tests;
• activities of daily living;
• overall response as reflected by global assessment.

Studies should stipulate two primary variables, one of which must evaluate cognition. For a claim of short-term treatment, responders may be defined at 6 months as improved to a relevant degree in cognition and not worsened in the two other domains.

The CPMP accepts that improvement in behavioural symptoms is important and that specific studies should be designed to assess this, but makes no detailed recommendations. It also accepts that cognitive improvement may be less relevant than functional or global improvement in more advanced disease.

The FDA also requires trials to show drug-related cognitive improvement as well as an overall effect which is determined by an independent physician (global functioning). Activities of daily living and behaviour are considered to be of secondary importance.

Cognitive impairment

Impairments in memory plus at least one other cognitive domain such as language, praxis, perceptual skills, problem-solving abilities, attention or orientation are essential for a formal diagnosis of 'probable AD'. Whilst memory may not always be the first area affected in 'possible AD' or other dementias, some impairment in cognition is expected.

Neuropsychological testing in dementia effectively began with the Blessed Dementia Scale. Developed to provide a quantitative measure of dementia, a link was demonstrated between the clinical effects of dementia and the degree of neuropathological change [4]. The scale also incorporated an Information–Memory–Concentration (IMC) test.

Cognitive assessments

Abbreviated Mental Test Score

The Abbreviated Mental Test Score (AMTS) [5] (Table 3.1) is a short form of a test derived from the Blessed Dementia Scale. It takes less than 5 min to do and is widely used in the UK by geriatricians and

Table 3.1 The Abbreviated Mental Test Score (AMTS)

1 Age
2 Time (to the nearest hour)
3 Repeat back an address (42 West Street) to be recalled at the end of the test
4 Year
5 Name of this place
6 Recognition of two people (doctor, nurse, . . .)
7 Date of birth
8 Dates of the First World War
9 Name of the present monarch
10 Count backwards from 20 to 1

Each question scores one mark; a score of 7 or 8 is suggested as the cut-off between cognitive impairment and normality.

general practitioners. It is almost exclusively a test of memory but is acceptable as a simple screening tool, for example in primary care. It can usefully be incorporated into an annual health screen such as is supposed to be offered to everyone in the UK over 75. People scoring full marks are unlikely to have significant dementia whilst those scoring less than 8 out of 10 should be investigated further.

The AMTS is not suitable as an outcome measure in clinical trials or for monitoring therapeutic response to a prescribed antidementia drug because it is insensitive. The two main measures that are used for these purposes are the Alzheimer's Disease Assessment Scale—Cognitive subscale (ADAS-Cog) and the Mini Mental State Examination (MMSE).

Alzheimer's Disease Assessment Scale and Alzheimer's Disease Assessment Scale-Cognitive

The ADAS [6] was developed to allow effective measurement of disease progression and the consequences of drug treatment for AD. Although independently measuring both cognitive and non-cognitive function, it is the ADAS-Cog that has been most widely used in clinical studies (Table 3.2).

The ADAS was designed to measure all major AD symptoms, to be reliable and relatively brief, to measure increases in symptom severity with disease progression, and to be suitable for use in a variety of settings (e.g. across cultures and languages). Versions are available for example in English, French, German, Spanish, Italian and Finnish, and other languages are in development. It is a performance-based scale that includes 11 items to assess cognitive function.

The ADAS-Cog score is an error score that can range from 0 (no errors) to a maximum of 70 (profoundly demented). Normal subjects score below 8–10 with very few people making no errors. It therefore

Table 3.2 The structure of the Alzheimer's Disease Assessment Scale–Cognitive (ADAS-Cog)

Domain	Number of items	Maximum error score
Memory	3	27
Orientation	1	8
Language	5	25
Praxis	2	10
Cognitive total	**11**	**70**

covers the full range of subjects without major ceiling or floor effects (although at high error scores the test becomes of little clinical value).

The scale has often been misunderstood because it is an error score with higher scores indicating poorer function. Most notably this occurred in the UK evidence-based medicine journal *Bandolier* that criticized a donepezil study yet failed to understand the ADAS-Cog, the main outcome measure [7].

Another source of misunderstanding is how a change in ADAS-Cog should be interpreted. Evidence from a US longitudinal study [8] showed that the average change in ADAS-Cog over 1 year for untreated AD patients was 9.55 ($\pm$ 8.21) points. However, the change can vary from some patients who deteriorate rapidly whilst others show little alteration in score. Moderately impaired people appeared to show a greater annual rate of change (13 points) than either mildly (6 points) or severely (7 points) impaired subjects.

The ADAS-Cog usually takes about 45 min to administer but it is not a timed test. It has been shown to be valid in clinical trials with significant drug–placebo differences for a number of cholinesterase inhibitors and several other compounds. Although not a requirement of regulatory authorities, it has become the standard cognitive assessment and a primary outcome of most recent clinical trials. It is not appropriate for routine use by non-specialists.

Mini Mental State Examination

The MMSE [9] is the most widely used brief measure of cognitive function and is appropriate for intermittent routine use. It has become the standard screening instrument for detecting cognitive impairment in elderly people and is available in several languages [10]. Often used as a secondary outcome measure in clinical trials, it is also acceptable as a brief assessment for following patients prescribed antidementia drugs. An annual deterioration of 3–4 points has been reported for untreated patients with AD. If a linear rate of disease progression is assumed, then patients would be expected to decline by 1–2 points over a 6-month period, the usual duration for the pivotal clinical trials in AD.

Interview based, it takes 10–15 min (see Table 3.3). Scores range from 0 (lowest) to 30 and the areas assessed are: orientation to time and place (10 points), registration of three words (3 points), attention and calculation (5 points), word recall (3 points), language (8 points) and visual construction (1 point). Areas not assessed include long-term memory and executive function.

Table 3.3 An example of the Mini Mental State Examination (MMSE)

Orientation

What day of the week is it today?	0/1
What month are we in?	0/1
What is today's date?	0/1
What year are we in?	0/1
What season of the year is it?	0/1
What town are we in?	0/1
What county (or state/province) are we in?	0/1
What country are we in?	0/1
Can you tell me the name of this place?	0/1
What floor of the building are we on?	0/1

Registration

Repeat until the person remembers three unrelated objects, e.g. ball, flag, tree (score after 1 trial, but repeat if necessary up to 5 trials)	0/3

Attention and calculation

Subtract 7 from 100 and keep subtracting until told to stop. Score after 5 subtractions. Spell the word 'world' forwards and ask the subject to spell it backwards 'DLROW'. Score letters in correct position. Enter higher of the two scores	0/5

Recall

What were the three words that you were asked to remember?	0/3

Naming

What is this called? (show a watch)	0/1
What is this called? (show a pencil)	0/1

Repetition

Repeat after me: 'No ifs, ands or buts'	0/1

Three-stage command

Take this paper in your left hand (or right, if left-handed), fold it in half with both hands and put it on the floor	0/3

Written command

Do what is written on this paper: 'close your eyes'	0/1

Writing

Write a short sentence	0/1

Copying

Copy this drawing (two intersecting pentagons). All 10 angles must be present and the intersection should form a quadrangle	0/1

Total score	**Maximum 30**

There has been considerable debate about how it should be performed and scored. There are no parallel forms although alternative words can be chosen for the registration/recall items (apple, table and penny are usually used but other words have included ball, flag, tree, shirt, brown, honesty, lemon, key and balloon). For attention and calculation, serial 7s are generally used but the alternate is to spell 'world' backwards (although deciding the score out of 5 is not always obvious). Many people now use both elements, taking the higher of the scores. Different items are frequently used for orientation to place, partly dependent on where the subject is tested.

Performance on the MMSE is influenced by educational level. In general, the sensitivity and specificity suggest that it is a valuable screening instrument for dementia and delirium. For subjects with more than 8 years of education, a score of 23 or less is usually indicative of cognitive impairment. Of course, no test should be used by itself to diagnose dementia.

Three levels are suggested: 24–30 = no cognitive impairment; 18–23 = mild to moderate impairment; and 17 or below = severe impairment. Intelligent patients may have a significant problem even though scoring 24 or above; patients with marked language impairment may score poorly suggesting that they are more severe than they actually are.

A number of suggestions have been made to modify the MMSE and a standardized version [11] may prove to be an improvement particularly for use in multicentre research studies.

Clock-drawing test

Clock drawing has been used for some years as a screening test for cognitive impairment and dementia. There are many ways of carrying out the test and normal clock-drawing ability reasonably excludes cognitive impairment. It is a useful adjunct to the MMSE or AMTS and is easy to record in clinical records to document change over time. It has also been used to follow the response to cholinesterase inhibitors.

The test requires verbal understanding, memory and spatially coded knowledge in addition to constructive skills [12]. A standard method is to ask the patient to draw a clock face marking the hours and then to set the hands at a particular time (e.g. 10 min past 11). Various scoring methods have been suggested. Using a 6-point scale is sufficient with 0 for no real attempt, 1 for an approximately circular face, 2 for the symmetry of number placement, 3 for the correctness of numbers, 4 for the presence of two hands and 5 for their correct time setting.

Activities of daily living

With the gradual decline in cognitive function, there are accompanying changes in performance of everyday activities. This impairment in social and occupational functioning is necessary for a formal (DSM-IV) diagnosis of dementia and also has a profound effect on the ability of the patient to live independently and safely. Any improvement in activities of daily living (ADL) is likely to be of benefit to the patient and their family as well as having a marked effect on quality of life.

ADL can be divided into two main types: basic activities of self-care (sometimes termed physical self-maintenance) which include feeding, dressing, bathing and toileting, and instrumental activities of daily living (IADL) which include more complex activities such as shopping, dealing with finances, looking after the home, and using transport. Complex activities are affected first in dementia with basic activities affected at a later stage.

Most patients in clinical trials are at a stage where basic ADLs are well preserved so that changes with drug treatment are best sought by the improved performance of IADLs. This is not easy because there are few scales that are both practical and suitable for this purpose. Older clinical trials usually used the Instrumental Activities of Daily Living (IADL)/Physical Self-Maintenance Scale (PSMS) that were not developed for use in dementia. Most current instruments have been developed specifically for dementia and have tried to remove any gender bias from the items evaluated as well as structuring the interview with the carer.

Assessment of activities of daily living

Progressive Deterioration Scale

The Progressive Deterioration Scale (PDS) [13] is a caregiver-rated measure that assesses quality of life changes or ADL on some 27 items. Scores range from 0 to 100 with lower scores indicating poorer performance. It assesses:
• normal socializing and responsiveness;
• involvement in family finances, budgeting, etc.;
• awareness of time;
• remembering where things are;
• appropriate eating and dressing;
• hobbies and household chores;
• independent travel.

The PDS has been used as an outcome measure in clinical trials with tacrine and rivastigmine.

Interview for Deterioration in Daily Living Activities in Dementia

The Interview for Deterioration in Daily Living Activities in Dementia (IDDD) [14] consists of a 33-item structured interview consisting of self-care activities such as washing, dressing and eating, as well as more complex activity items such as shopping, writing and answering the telephone, activities performed equally by men and women. The frequency of assistance is rated on a 3-point scale for each item giving an overall score ranging from 33 (best) to 99 (worst).

The IDDD has been used in one of the pivotal trials with donepezil.

Disability Assessment for Dementia

This ADL rating takes about 20 min to complete either as a questionnaire completed by the caregiver or as a structured interview of the caregiver. It assesses the ability of the patient to initiate, plan, organize and perform basic (for example, eating) and more complex (for example, leisure and housework) instrumental ADL. The Disability Assessment for Dementia (DAD) [15] has been used in clinical trials involving metrifonate.

Global functioning

Assessment of global functioning allows a single subjective integrated judgement of the patient's symptoms and performance by a clinician experienced in the management of AD patients. It represents a way to validate results obtained in comprehensive scales or objective tests [2].

Clinicians' global assessments can be divided into those that assess the severity of dementia and those that assess change. For some assessments, there is an assumption that dementia progresses in an orderly, linear way. This is clearly too simplistic but it is helpful to identify whether patients have mild, moderate or severe dementia. The two most frequently used severity scales are also increasingly being used to measure subjects with milder problems than dementia (e.g. questionable dementia, mild cognitive impairment or age-related cognitive decline).

Global interview-based severity scales

These scales can be useful at the initial assessment or review of patients attending, for example, a memory clinic. They are also useful to follow changes in severity within the clinical trials setting and will become increasingly relevant for demonstrating delay in the progression of dementia by disease-modifying drugs. The two most widely used scales are the Clinical Dementia Rating (CDR) Scale and the Global Deterioration Scale (GDS); both use anchor points to guide the rater.

Clinical Dementia Rating Scale

The CDR [16] is an old scale first described in 1982. Based on a comprehensive structured interview using worksheets, most of the information will have been collected as part of a normal clinical clerking. Its main characteristics are:
- structured interview with patient and an informant requiring about 40 min;
- six domains are assessed: memory, orientation, judgement and problem-solving, community activities, home and hobbies, and personal care;
- 5-point scale with 0 for no impairment, 0.5 for questionable dementia and 1, 2, 3 for mild, moderate and severe dementia, respectively.

The scoring has been updated more recently [17] with an aggregate rating based on the Sum of Boxes, each box based on performance within a given domain.

The CDR is currently the gold standard global severity rating for clinical trials in AD. This is mainly because, using the Sum of Boxes approach, the criteria for a given rating have been better operationalized to encourage more uniformity across different centres and raters.

Global Deterioration Scale

Also described in 1982, the GDS [18] has stood the test of time too. Unlike the CDR it is not based on a structured interview but on information gathered as part of the routine clinical assessment. Its main characteristics are:
- takes less than 5 min (once general information collected);
- assesses severity according to cognitive, functional and behavioural domains;
- 7-point scale of severity or stage of dementia with 1 = normal, 2 = normal ageing/age-related cognitive decline, 3 = mild cognitive

impairment/incipient AD, 4 = mild AD, 5 = moderate AD, 6 = moderately severe AD, 7 = severe late AD (requires continuous assistance).

The GDS is well validated and more sensitive to change than the MMSE. Like the CDR it is probably relatively free of educational, cultural, occupational and other biases.

By combining the GDS with another assessment, the Functional Assessment Staging (FAST) [19], it is possible to subdivide GDS 6 and 7 into 11 substages that allow a more detailed categorization of people with severe dementia. Although of little relevance at present with current drug treatments, this may become more important in the future as disease-modifying treatments are developed.

Global interview-based change scales

Clinical global ratings of change have been used in psychopharmacology for many years. The 'Clinician's Global Assessment' was one of the two outcome measures that the FDA identified as essential to the assessment of efficacy of antidementia drugs in clinical trials [3]. The FDA initially emphasized that this rating should be based only on changes in behaviour personally observed/assessed by the clinician. This unrealistic view seems to have been partly driven by the fear that knowledge, for example of side-effects, would unblind the observer (and this would have been likely with tacrine that was being evaluated at the time of these decisions).

Clinical Global Impressions of Change (CGIC) are global ratings that are made after interviewing the patient and often the principal caregiver. The underlying construct assumes that if drug effects are meaningful there will be changes in the patient that are obvious to an experienced clinical observer.

Early scales were mostly unstructured with poor inter-rater reliability and they appeared insensitive to drug effects. More recent CGIC have increased the measure's structure but they have often not been properly validated.

The rating can be carried out by an experienced physician, clinical psychologist or nurse; the caregiver should be interviewed separately; and some formal assessment of mental status is helpful but must not dominate the assessment of the patient which is best guided by a set of similar questions or worksheets.

All CGIC are intended to be holistic and to determine how the patient is by comparison with a detailed baseline assessment. The global rater should by definition be relatively independent of other study activity.

Ratings are made on a 7-point scale where 4 = no change; 5, 6 and 7 represent increasing degrees of deterioration; and 3, 2 and 1 increasing degrees of improvement.

A number of variations have been or are being used in trials with antidementia compounds. They include the FDA Clinicians' Interview-Based Impression of Change (CIBIC) that only interviews the patient; the CIBIC-Plus where an informant is interviewed as well; the CIBI, developed by Parke-Davis Pharmaceuticals in cooperation with the US FDA and used in a major 30-week study of tacrine that contributed significantly to its approval by the FDA; and the US AD Cooperative Study Clinical Global Impression of Change (ADCS-CGIC) that assesses 15 areas under the domains of cognition, behaviour, social and daily functionings. There is still discussion about whether the patient or the informant should be interviewed first. For any given study, the same order must be used by all sites and raters.

Assessment of behavioural and psychological problems

Although cognitive impairment is the most consistent feature of AD and other dementias, it is the psychiatric and behavioural disturbances that are of most importance and distress to the patient and caregiver. Patients in clinical trials are unlikely to suffer with major behavioural problems because the protocol usually excludes subjects with significant depression or psychotic features that require medication such as antidepressants or neuroleptics. However, assessing behaviour has become more important because clinical trials are lasting longer, often 12 months or more, especially in open-label extension studies. Also, it has become clear that cholinergic drugs do modify certain aspects of behaviour. Finally, regulatory authorities like the CPMP have suggested that clinical trials should be carried out specifically to assess behavioural effects (and, for example, this has now been done with risperidone—see Chapter 5).

The scales that are most relevant to drug evaluation in clinical trials are discussed in the following sections. They rate the frequency and/or severity of behaviours, usually requiring a caregiver or the physician to make the rating.

Alzheimer's Disease Assessment Scale—Non-cognitive

The ADAS was originally designed to evaluate all aspects of AD [6]. In some trials, the ADAS-Cog and ADAS-Non-cognitive (Noncog) have

both been included as primary outcome measures. More recently, the ADAS-Noncog has been less popular and replaced by other scales. Its characteristics are:
• assesses 10 non-cognitive features: tearfulness,* depression,* concentration, uncooperativeness, delusions,* hallucinations,* pacing,* motor activity,* tremors, and appetite* (items marked with an asterisk include report on previous 7 days, other items rated by the tester based on behaviour during ADAS-Cog);
• marked on a 6-point scale (0 = not present, to 5 = severe); scores range from 50 (most severe) to 0 and can be combined with ADAS-Cog to give a total score.

Behavioural Pathology in Alzheimer's Disease Scale

The Behavioural Pathology in Alzheimer's Disease Scale (BEHAVE-AD) [20] is probably the earliest behaviour rating scale in AD and was intended for use in studies of behavioural symptoms and in pharmacological trials. Its characteristics are:
• rating done by a clinician and takes 20 min;
• assesses 25 well-defined behaviours in seven areas: paranoid and delusional ideation, hallucinations, activity disturbances, aggressiveness, diurnal rhythm disturbances, affective disturbances and anxieties/phobias;
• refers to the 2 weeks before the interview and involves an informed caregiver;
• behaviour, if present, rated as mild, moderate or severe.

Neuropsychiatric Inventory

The Neuropsychiatric Inventory (NPI) [21] is an efficient scale that is being increasingly used by pharmaceutical companies to assess the effects of drugs on psychiatric symptoms and behaviour in patients with AD and other dementias. Its main characteristics are:
• structured interview with the caregiver taking 15–30 min;
• assesses 12 behaviours on the basis of frequency (0 = absent, to 4 = at least daily) and severity (1–3) giving score from 0 to 144 (maximum);
• also often assesses carer's distress (0–5) as a result of the behaviour.
    Areas covered include delusions, hallucinations, agitation/aggression, depression/dysphoria, anxiety, elation/euphoria, apathy/indifference, disinhibition, irritability/lability, aberrant motor behaviour, sleep, and appetite and eating disorders.

Quality of life

There is a significant school of thought [22] that emphasizes that people with dementia are people first and foremost and that there is much that can be done in a general way to improve their quality of life while waiting for the 'magic bullets' of medical science. This view is one that should not be forgotten.

Quality of life (QOL) is a very difficult area to discuss in the context of antidementia drug therapy. It is difficult enough to measure in people without cognitive impairment. However, obtaining a reliable assessment of a patient's own QOL and comparing whether it has improved or not during a clinical trial lasting 6 months or more is unlikely in the presence of significant memory problems. It is also important to be clear whose QOL is being assessed: is it the patient's or is it the carer's?

A patient's scale was adapted for use in clinical trials with donepezil as an attempt to look at QOL. It was totally unsatisfactory and did not give positive results yet left the company open to unfair criticism that the drug did not affect QOL. The CPMP guidelines [2] acknowledge this issue stating that 'although QOL is an important dimension of the consequences of diseases, the lack of validation of its assessment in AD does not allow specific recommendations to be made as yet'.

At present, improvements in QOL for patients and/or carers can only be inferred from scales for behaviour and global change combined with a more general evaluation. The PDS, described above, is an ADL measure that has also been identified as a QOL measure that may be promising.

Limitations of current assessment scales

The problem with QOL assessment is a useful reminder that although rating scales are helpful and necessary both in research and in clinical practice, they must not be overvalued.

The assessments most widely used in dementia drug trials are generally those developed partly or mainly in response to regulatory requirements. This is not always ideal and may discourage development of better assessments or assessments for areas not covered by the regulations (this is illustrated by the later introduction of scales such as the NPI that assess behavioural problems). However, it is essential for drug companies if they want to maximize the chances of getting a particular drug through the regulatory hoops. For the consumer this is clearly vital. An unlicensed therapy is an unavailable therapy no matter how many peer-reviewed publications there are supporting its efficacy.

Critics have often complained that the effects of current drug therapy are small or of little significance. These criticisms are often based on mean changes in scores such as the ADAS-Cog. There is considerable heterogeneity among people with AD or other dementing disorders. When comparing the mean differences in rating scales between patients on drug treatment and those on placebo, it is important to remember that individual patients may do considerably better (or worse) than the average. For an incurable, terminal illness like dementia, those doing significantly better than the average should not be overlooked.

There is increasing interest in trying to define responders to drug therapy in an attempt to overcome some of these difficulties. Regulatory authorities appear to have defined a clinically significant response as an improvement of at least 4 points on the ADAS-Cog particularly if accompanied by an improvement (score < 4) on a global rating such as the CIBIC-Plus or at least no deterioration on the CIBIC-Plus and the ADL assessment. A 4-point decline on ADAS-Cog is roughly the decline expected in untreated patients over 6 months, although, as will be seen from Chapter 4, placebo groups in clinical trials have often shown a smaller decline than this.

References

1 Orrell M, Woods B. Tacrine and psychological therapies in dementia—no contest? *Int J Geriatr Psychiatry* 1996; 11: 189–92.

2 Committee for Proprietary Medicinal Products (CPMP). *Note for Guidance on Medicinal Products in the Treatment of Alzheimer's Disease.* London: EMEA, 1997.

3 Leber P. *Guidelines for the Clinical Evaluation of Anti-Dementia Drugs,* 1st Draft. Rockville MD: US Food and Drug Administration, 1990.

4 Blessed G, Tomlinson BE, Roth M. The association between quantitative measures of dementia and of senile changes in the cerebral gray matter of elderly subjects. *Br J Psychiatry* 1968; 114: 797–811.

5 Hodkinson HM. Evaluation of a mental test score for assessment of mental impairment in the elderly. *Age Ageing* 1972; 1: 233–8.

6 Rosen WG, Mohs RG, Davis KL. A new rating scale for Alzheimer's disease. *Am J Psychiatry* 1984; 141: 1356–64.

7 Anonymous. New dementia drug. *Bandolier* 1997; 40: 2–5.

8 Stern RG, Mohs RC, Davidson M *et al.* A longitudinal study of Alzheimer's disease: measurement, rate, and predictors of cognitive deterioration. *Am J Psychiatry* 1994; 151: 390–6.

9 Folstein MF, Folstein SE, McHugh PR. 'Mini-Mental State': a practical method for grading the cognitive state of patients for the clinician. *J Psychiatr Res* 1975; 12: 189–98.

10 Tombaugh TN, McIntyre NJ. The Mini-Mental State Examination: a comprehensive review. *J Am Geriatr Soc* 1992; 40: 922–35.

11 Molloy DW, Alemayehu E, Roberts R. Reliability of a Standardized Mini-Mental State Examination compared with the traditional Mini-Mental State Examination. *Am J Psychiatry* 1991; 148: 102–5.

12 Agrell B, Dehlin O. The clock-drawing test. *Age Ageing* 1998; 27: 399–403.

13 DeJong R, Osterlund OW, Roy GW. Measurement of quality-of-life changes in patients with Alzheimer's disease. *Clin Ther* 1989; 11: 545–54.

14 Teunisse S, Derix MMA, van Crevel H. Assessing the severity of dementia: patient and caregiver. *Arch Neurol* 1991; 48: 274–7.

15 Gelinas I, Auer S. Functional autonomy. In: Gauthier S, ed. *Clinical Diagnosis and Management of Alzheimer's Disease.* London: Martin Dunitz, 1996: 191–9.

16 Hughes CP, Berg L, Danziger WL, Coben LA, Martin RL. A new clinical scale for the staging of dementia. *Br J Psychiatry* 1982; 140: 566–72.

17 Morris JC. The CDR: current version and scoring rules. *Neurology* 1993; 43: 2412–14.

18 Reisberg B, Ferris SH, deLeon MJ, Crook T. The global deterioration scale for assessment of primary degenerative dementia. *Am J Psychiatry* 1982; 139: 1136–9.

19 Reisberg B. Functional assessment staging (FAST). *Psychopharmacol Bull* 1988; 24: 653–9.

20 Reisberg B, Borenstein J, Salob SP, Ferris SH, Franssen E, Georgotas A. Behavioural symptoms in Alzheimer's disease: phenomenology and treatment. *J Clin Psychiatry* 1987; 48 (Suppl. 5): 9–15.

21 Cummings JL, Mega M, Gray K, Rosenberg-Thompson S, Carusi DA, Gornbein J. The Neuropsychiatric Inventory: comprehensive assessment of psychopathology in dementia. *Neurology* 1994; 44: 2308–14.

22 Kitwood T. *Dementia Reconsidered: the Person Comes First.* Buckingham: Open University Press, 1997.

4 Antidementia drugs

Over the past 30 years many compounds have been considered for potential use in the treatment of Alzheimer's disease (AD) and other dementias. The previous chapter has considered the various symptoms or symptom complexes that can potentially be targeted with drug treatment.

The dementias produce specific abnormalities in memory and cognition. Antidementia drug therapy has been targeted at these symptoms but has usually been developed for AD rather than for dementias in general. This chapter will consider the various approaches to improving intellectual function.

So far the most successful pharmacological strategy has been the manipulation of the cholinergic system using acetylcholinesterase inhibitors. Four are already licensed in some countries and several others have been submitted for approval or are in clinical trials. Treatments acting more directly on muscarinic and nicotinic receptors or involving other neurotransmitters and growth factors may lead to even more effective therapies. In addition, there are several alternatives that depend on our current understanding of the pathological changes that lead to dementia. Knowledge of these changes has developed dramatically over the last few years.

Replacing acetylcholine

The cholinergic hypothesis is discussed in Chapter 1 (p. 6). Abnormalities in the cholinergic system appear to be a particularly significant and consistent feature of AD and some other dementias. Replacement of acetylcholine has been shown to be beneficial but is likely only to provide symptomatic therapy (see Box 4.1). There have been suggestions that this approach may also have the potential to alter the disease process. This has some theoretical support with recent information

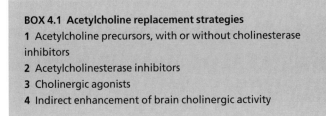

BOX 4.1 Acetylcholine replacement strategies
1 Acetylcholine precursors, with or without cholinesterase inhibitors
2 Acetylcholinesterase inhibitors
3 Cholinergic agonists
4 Indirect enhancement of brain cholinergic activity

that cholinergic receptor activation may alter processing of the amyloid precursor protein, APP.

Acetylcholine precursors

Supplementation with precursors like choline and lecithin has been tried in several studies, often giving heroic doses. Since there is more choline in the cerebrospinal fluid (CSF) of patients with AD than in controls, and choline levels increase with disease progression, these approaches may not be logical; it may be that the problem is choline uptake rather than the amount available. Most studies have failed to show significant benefit and this approach has largely been abandoned.

Early clinical trials with the cholinesterase inhibitor tacrine combined its administration with lecithin but this is unnecessary.

Acetylcholinesterase inhibitors

There are two main types of cholinesterase in the brain, acetylcholinesterase and butyrylcholinesterase [1]. Acetylcholinesterase is the predominant enzyme and exists in several forms. The extracellular G4 form is most abundant in the brain but there is also a smaller amount of the intracellular G1 form. In AD it is the G4 form that appears to be most reduced.

Acetylcholinesterase has been detected in senile plaques and neurofibrillary tangles. Butyrylcholinesterase activity also appears to be increased in AD brain although its function in the brain is unclear. Acetylcholinesterase activity can be measured in erythrocytes while butyrylcholinesterase (pseudo or non-specific cholinesterase) is found in serum.

The acetylcholinesterase inhibitors that have been evaluated in AD are structurally different with different relative specificities for acetylcholinesterase and butyrylcholinesterase. This may give them slightly different profiles of efficacy and adverse effects; they may also show different subsidiary activities that may be clinically relevant. So far, the subsidiary activities have been studied in more detail with tacrine [1] than with other compounds.

Tacrine (Cognex; Parke-Davis)

In 1993, tacrine (also called tetrahydroaminoacridine or THA) became the first agent approved specifically for treating the cognitive symptoms of AD.

Pharmacology

Mode of action

Tacrine is a centrally active, non-competitive reversible inhibitor of acetylcholinesterase and butyrylcholinesterase. In patients receiving tacrine hydrochloride 160 mg/day, the highest recommended clinical dose, red blood cell acetylcholinesterase was inhibited by 60% and plasma cholinesterase by 40%. The drug has other pharmacological activity including effects on monoamine levels, binding to muscarinic and nicotinic receptors, and blocking of sodium and potassium channels. It has been suggested that some of these properties might be relevant to the clinical effects of the compound [2].

Pharmacokinetics

The pharmacokinetic parameters for tacrine show wide inter-individual variation. Oral bioavailability ranges from 17 to 37% with peak plasma levels reached in 1–2 h. Food decreases the rate and extent of absorption. It is extensively metabolized in the liver, and the major metabolite, 1-hydroxytacrine (velnacrine), is clinically active on its own. The elimination half-life for tacrine is 1.3–7 h in patients with AD [1]. There is a positive correlation between tacrine plasma concentrations and the degree of cholinesterase inhibition in plasma.

Clinical evidence

Efficacy

A systematic review evaluated 21 published trials [3], lasting 3–36 weeks, which were randomized and placebo controlled.

There were 3555 patients with mild to moderate AD who commenced treatment. Tacrine showed a modest improvement in cognitive function and in functional ability in just over 20% of patients at 3–6 months of treatment. Cognitive improvement was defined as a 3–4-point improvement in the Alzheimer's Disease Assessment Scale—Cognitive (ADAS-Cog) and 2–3 points in the Mini Mental State Examination (MMSE). This is on average equivalent to about 6–12 months' delay in the cognitive deterioration that would normally be expected in AD and is considered clinically relevant by the US Food and Drug Administration (FDA) [3].

A second systematic review has conducted a meta-analysis with central analysis of individual patient data using the Cochrane Dementia Group registry of trials [4]. This analysis included information from 12 double-blind trials completed before January 1996 involving 1984 patients. Tacrine reduced deterioration in cognitive function during the first 3 months and increased the odds of global cognitive improvement. Effects on behavioural disturbance as assessed by the ADAS-Noncog were of uncertain clinical significance. Functional autonomy was not significantly improved but the data available were limited. There was a suggestion that benefit was greater with higher doses (120–160 mg).

Tacrine has also been shown to improve behavioural symptoms in AD, sometimes independently of cognitive response, supporting a cholinergic basis for some of these problems [5] (see Chapter 5, p. 78).

The results of one study [6] showed that patients who remained on tacrine doses greater than 80 mg/day in the longer term (minimum follow-up 2 years) were less likely to have entered a nursing home than patients on lower doses or who discontinued the drug.

Adverse events

In the larger systematic review [3] withdrawal was high at about one-third of patients, with over 80% being tacrine-related. Data from the individual patient meta-analysis [4] suggest that one patient withdrew for every four patients treated.

Adverse events affected about 60% of patients of which about one-third were due to cholinergic side-effects and one-third due to elevated liver transaminases [3]. Cholinergic side-effects, seen to varying degrees with all cholinesterase inhibitors, mainly consist of gastrointestinal symptoms, including nausea, vomiting and diarrhoea, sweating, and bradycardia; headache and myalgia have also been reported. Adverse events were more frequent at doses over 100 mg and disappeared on discontinuation of tacrine. They usually occur soon after initiation of treatment or when the dose is increased.

The frequent liver function abnormalities are due to a specific reversible hepatotoxicity that appears to be particular to tacrine (and its clinically active metabolite, 1-hydroxytacrine [HP029, velnacrine]) as an aminoacridine. The median onset of abnormal liver function tests is at 6 weeks. Patients with elevated transaminases can be rechallenged with the drug and around two-thirds will get no further problem even if given higher doses than before [1].

Practical use

Indications

Symptomatic treatment of mild to moderate AD.

Dosage and administration

The initial dosage of tacrine is 10 mg four times daily and this is increased every 4–6 weeks to a maximum of 40 mg four times daily; efficacy is likely to be greatest if patients are titrated to the maximum tolerated dose. Regular monitoring of serum transaminases is essential particularly during the titration period or if the dose is subsequently increased.

Place of tacrine in the management of Alzheimer's disease

The efficacy of tacrine in mild to moderate AD is clear and consistent and of benefit to some 30–40% of those who can tolerate it. Response appears to be related to dose (with the best results at doses of 120–160 mg/day) but tolerability and especially the hepatotoxicity have limited its usefulness. In addition it needs to be taken frequently and this is another limitation in predominantly elderly patients with memory problems.

In general, tacrine has been displaced by its successors, donepezil and rivastigmine.

Availability

An aminoacridine compound, it became widely used in many countries including the USA, Sweden and France but has never been marketed in the UK.

Donepezil (Aricept; Eisai/Pfizer)

The year of 1997 saw the approval of donepezil, the first drug to be marketed in the UK for the symptomatic treatment of mild or moderate dementia in AD.

Pharmacology

Mode of action

Donepezil is a piperidine-based reversible inhibitor of acetylcholinesterase, chemically distinct from tacrine. It is highly selective for acetylcholinesterase with much less activity against butyrylcholinesterase, an enzyme mainly present outside the central nervous system (CNS). Red blood cell acetylcholinesterase inhibition at steady state was 64% with 5 mg/day and 77% with 10 mg/day. Inhibition up to 90% has been reported during long-term treatment with 10 mg/day [1].

Pharmacokinetics

Absorption is complete with peak plasma concentrations being reached in 3–4 h. The elimination half-life is long (70–80 h) and steady-state plasma levels are reached after about 15 days. Neither food nor time of administration (morning or evening) influences the rate or extent of absorption.

The drug is approximately 95% protein-bound. It is metabolized in the liver by enzymes of the cytochrome P450 system. In theory this might suggest a potential for interactions with other compounds that act through this system (e.g. erythromycin, itraconazole, fluoxetine and enzyme inducers such as rifampicin). Studies with warfarin, digoxin and cimetidine have not shown any problem. However, the summary of product characteristics advises caution since it may be that all possible interactions have not yet been recorded.

Clinical evidence

Efficacy

Data submitted for registration came from three randomized controlled trials involving over 1100 patients in the USA over 14–30 weeks. Several studies have now been published together with the results from a large European multinational study involving 818 patients which also confirms efficacy. Many patients in the controlled trials have continued into open-label extension studies and have received donepezil for periods in excess of 2 years.

The key study involved 473 patients and compared once-daily doses of 5 or 10 mg with placebo given for 24 weeks [7]. The primary endpoints were to show improvement on the ADAS-Cog and the overall global effect using the Clinicians' Interview-Based Impression of Change (CIBIC)-Plus. The CIBIC-Plus used was a semistructured instrument intended to examine four major areas of patient function: general, cognitive, behavioural and activities of daily living.

There were significant improvements in both primary assessments. Some 26% of patients receiving 10 mg improved by 7 points or more on the ADAS-Cog (in comparison with 8% on placebo) which equates to at least 6–12-month gain in cognitive function compared with baseline. On the CIBIC-Plus, only 1 in 10 patients on placebo improved in contrast with 1 in 4 patients receiving donepezil. Regulatory authorities are interested in responder analyses such as the number needed to treat (NNT) and at a 4-point change in ADAS-Cog. At 10 mg/day, the NNT for this is only 4 (i.e. four patients would need to be treated to see such an improvement in one patient) whilst the NNT for improvement on the CIBIC is 8 [8].

After the double-blind phase, all patients entered a 6-week placebo washout. At the end of this, the drug treatment groups were indistinguishable from the original placebo group suggesting that the benefits are symptomatic with no effect on the disease process.

Open-label data for 2 years or more show a gradual deterioration after 26 weeks' total treatment time [9]. However, the average ADAS-Cog score of the patients remained above their entry score until week 50 (i.e. as a group their cognitive function was improved for this time). The rate of change in ADAS-Cog score from week 26 was 6.6 points per year, comparable with that previously reported for untreated patients. This suggests a continued treatment effect with long-term therapy that is also confirmed by more general clinical use [10].

Anecdotally, some patients clearly show an improvement that is more remarkable and sustained than the group data might suggest. This is not surprising and illustrates the danger of basing all judgements about a therapy on mean data and forgetting about the individual patient. In some patients, the benefits are so obvious that formal evaluation is almost superfluous.

A Cochrane review [11] has assessed the main trials and concluded that there are modest improvements in cognitive function and global clinical effect. Data from the trials have now been supported by data from typical clinical practice [12]. There was clinically meaningful improvement in cognitive function and a reduction in neuropsychiatric symptoms in nearly 40% of patients associated with reduced carer distress. Continued benefit on ADAS-Cog was seen in responders for up to 15 months.

A further double-blind placebo-controlled study has evaluated efficacy over 1 year [13]. Cognition was maintained at or near baseline with donepezil and this was significantly better than with placebo. There was also a significant difference for activities of daily living (ADL) and global function.

Adverse events

Despite being specific for acetylcholinesterase, the side-effects of donepezil are typical for this class of compound and include diarrhoea, muscle cramps, fatigue, nausea, vomiting, insomnia and dizziness. They are generally mild and transient, occur early in the course of treatment, and often resolve in a few days despite continued therapy. As with similar drugs, caution should be observed when prescribing in the presence of bradycardia and atrial or ventricular conduction disorders.

Practical use

Indications

> The drug is indicated for the symptomatic treatment of mild or moderate dementia in AD.

Dosage and administration

> It has a simple dosing schedule starting with 5 mg once daily which may be increased to 10 mg after at least 1 month to reduce the risks of side-effects. It is recommended that it is given in the evening, presumably to minimize gastrointestinal side-effects. This may be impractical sometimes and can be ignored. Dosing in the morning can sometimes help those who develop insomnia with the drug. Benefits will not be seen in all patients (a provisional estimate is that about 40% of suitable patients will respond). Formal assessment using a test like the MMSE is important for aiding in the diagnosis of dementia and assessing the benefits of therapy. Patients with mild to moderate dementia will usually score more than 10 out of 30 on the MMSE.

Place of donepezil in the management of Alzheimer's disease

> In the USA donepezil rapidly replaced tacrine as the drug of choice. It is a once-daily dose compared with three or four times a day with tacrine. More importantly, it does not affect hepatic enzymes like tacrine does.

Availability

> Donepezil is undoubtedly an important step in the drug treatment of AD. It has now been approved in over 50 countries including the USA, Canada, Australia, New Zealand, much of Europe, South Africa and Japan, and is marketed in some 36 of these countries.

Rivastigmine (Exelon; Novartis)

Pharmacology

Mode of action

> Rivastigmine is a centrally selective carbamate inhibitor of acetylcholinesterase. It forms a carbamylated complex with the enzyme that inactivates it for about 10 h (despite itself having a short plasma half-life of 1–2 h) producing 'pseudo-irreversible' inhibition. It is described as 'brain selective' with particular activity in the cortex and hippocampus and preferentially inhibits the G1 form of acetylcholinesterase, a

form relatively more abundant in the brain in AD. A single 3-mg oral dose produces 30–40% inhibition of central acetylcholinesterase but minimal inhibition in the red cell or plasma. In contrast, it has been shown to inhibit both acetylcholinesterase and butyrylcholinesterase in the CSF to a similar extent [1].

Pharmacokinetics

No detailed pharmacokinetic data have been published. Some data in the product literature are confusing. Absorption is reported as rapid and complete yet bioavailability increases with dose. Administration of the drug with food slows absorption and increases the area under the concentration–time curve by about 30%. Absolute bioavailability after a 3-mg dose is reported as about $36 \pm 13\%$. Rivastigmine readily crosses the blood–brain barrier.

It is rapidly and extensively metabolized, primarily by liver cholinesterase-mediated hydrolysis, to a minimally active metabolite. This may then undergo *N*-demethylation and/or sulphate conjugation. The metabolite is eliminated rapidly by the kidney and unchanged drug is not found in the urine.

The weak protein binding (about 40%) and the absence of significant metabolism by hepatic microsomal (cytochrome P450) enzymes minimizes the risk of clinically relevant drug interactions, apart from with drugs acting directly on the cholinergic system.

Clinical evidence

Efficacy

The main efficacy studies with rivastigmine have been carried out within the international ADENA (Alzheimer's disease treatment with ENA-713 [rivastigmine] programme). This has involved over 3300 patients and is probably the largest formal clinical trial programme yet conducted for an antidementia treatment (although tacrine trials overall have involved more subjects).

Full data are not available from about half of the patients studied in trials to date and several large studies remain unpublished or published only in part. Reports from the ADENA programme do not make clear how missing data are replaced in intention-to-treat analyses and this could potentially exaggerate benefits of therapy [14].

Nevertheless, a systematic review [15] has been published of what appear to be three well-designed, adequately powered, 26-week clinical trials involving 2126 patients (1479 on rivastigmine and 647 on placebo). Memory and cognition were measured using the ADAS-Cog.

The clinician's global assessment of change was measured using the CIBIC-Plus. A pooled analysis showed that in doses of 6–12 mg/day rivastigmine demonstrated a consistent significant difference in efficacy compared with placebo. Rivastigmine 1–4 mg/day demonstrated some benefits over placebo but it was not as effective as higher doses. In the two main studies, there was also a significant improvement on an ADL scale at 6–12 mg/day.

In another pooled analysis of 945 patients, 21% of those receiving 6–12 mg/day rivastigmine improved cognitively on ADAS-Cog by at least 4 points in comparison with 12% on placebo (intention-to-treat analysis); only 10% were 'responders' when CIBIC-Plus and ADL were also considered in comparison to 6% on placebo [16]. The drug appears to have its greatest effects on symptoms associated with short-term memory loss [17]. Interestingly, rivastigmine appears to be more effective in patients 75 years or older and patients who are non-smokers.

In the first of the ADENA studies to be published [18], 235 patients were randomly assigned to placebo, 233 to relatively low doses of rivastigmine (1–4 mg/day) and 231 to higher doses (6–12 mg/day) for 26 weeks. There was an initial fixed dose-titration phase through week 7, followed by a flexible dose phase during weeks 8–26 when doses were increased within the assigned range until the maximum dose or maximum tolerated dose was achieved. A dose decrease was permitted providing the dose remained within the target range.

By the end of the study, the mean doses for patients in the 1–4 mg and 6–12 mg groups were 3.5 and 9.7 mg, respectively. By week 26, 83% of patients in the low-dose group were receiving 4 mg of rivastigmine and 55% in the high-dose group were receiving 12 mg.

Both dose regimens showed significant benefit for cognition, global functioning and severity (stage) of disease. The higher dose also produced significant benefit for ADL. On the ADAS-Cog, this study showed the largest drug vs. placebo difference that 'ha[s] been reported to date for a dementia drug (4.94 points)' [18]. This value is taken from the observed-cases analysis not the intention-to-treat analysis which is less (3.78 points). The difference is mainly represented by the deterioration on placebo (4.15 points); it is suggested that this results reflects the natural decline of patients with AD more closely than in studies with other compounds and may result from the more liberal inclusion criteria in the ADENA programme. Data from the other published ADENA study [19] with similar entry criteria show a much smaller decline in the placebo group (1.41 on the observed cases data and 1.34 on the intention-to-treat data) illustrating the difficulty of comparing data from different studies even with the same drug. (Differences have also been shown between the two main published studies for donepezil.)

Long-term efficacy and tolerability data for rivastigmine have not yet been published in detail but data from long-term open-label studies suggest that the benefits do continue. Even after 2 years, the cognitive decline on those receiving 6–12 mg/day was less than that in patients receiving placebo for 6 months in the above study [20]. This same report also notes that the drug is significantly more effective than placebo in patients with vascular risk factors suggesting potential for use in vascular dementia (VaD). There are also suggestions that it may be effective in patients with moderately severe and severe AD (based on the Global Deterioration Scale (GDS) severity score) including beneficial effects on behaviour [20].

Adverse events

Higher doses are associated with greater efficacy but also with an increased risk of adverse events. Despite a possibly more selective action, the adverse events are typical of cholinesterase inhibitors as a class. The most common (with an incidence of ≥ 5% and twice the frequency of placebo) were asthenia, anorexia, dizziness, somnolence and vomiting. As with donepezil these are often mild and transient and tend to occur on starting the drug or when increasing the dose. Female subjects were more susceptible to nausea, vomiting, loss of appetite and weight loss. As a result, the patient's weight should be monitored during therapy.

The occurrence of serious adverse events was similar to placebo but there were more withdrawals due to adverse events with the drug at doses of 6 mg/day or above (7.9% for placebo compared with 9.4, 14.9 and 17.5%, respectively, for 6, 9 and 12 mg/day). During the clinical trials more deaths occurred in the drug-treated group than on placebo, but the Committee for Proprietary Medicinal Products (CPMP) did not believe that the data indicated an increased mortality rate with rivastigmine.

As with other cholinomimetic agents including donepezil, care must be taken when using rivastigmine in patients with sick sinus syndrome or other conduction defects.

Practical use

Indications

Like donepezil, it is indicated for the symptomatic treatment of mild to moderate AD.

Dosage and administration

The drug is administered with food twice daily commencing at 1.5 mg b.d. and increasing at a minimum of 2-weekly intervals to achieve the effective dose range of 3–6 mg b.d.

Place of rivastigmine in the management of Alzheimer's disease

In general, the efficacy of rivastigmine seems similar to that of tacrine and donepezil. Based on the results of published trials, donepezil may be better tolerated than rivastigmine. Comparing trials may give a false picture of efficacy and tolerability because of the different populations used with different entry criteria and different comorbidities, and in the rivastigmine trials patients were often titrated to the highest tolerated dose. No direct comparisons of the two drugs have yet been made. Both are better tolerated than tacrine

Compared with donepezil, rivastigmine has to be given twice daily and dose-titration is more complex; this may be a disadvantage but there is more flexibility within this dosage regimen. Rivastigmine is generally cheaper than donepezil.

No data are available for switching patients from one drug to the other, either because of lack of efficacy or side-effects. It is reasonable to try both drugs if necessary.

Availability

In 1998, rivastigmine (Exelon) was approved and marketed in the European Community. It is also available in many other countries including Switzerland, Mexico, Argentina, Guatemala, Brazil, Peru, Ecuador, Trinidad and Tobago, Nicaragua, New Zealand, Thailand and Hong Kong. It will be launched in the USA in 2000.

Galantamine (galanthamine, Reminyl; Shire/Janssen-Cilag)

Galantamine is a phenanthrene alkaloid extracted from snowdrop and daffodil bulbs (*Galanthus nivalis*), although a synthetic process has now been developed.

Pharmacology

Mode of action

It is a reversible, competitive acetylcholinesterase inhibitor; 30–60% inhibition of red blood cell acetylcholinesterase is obtained 30–45 min after oral galantamine [1]. Activity against acetylcholinesterase is more than 50-fold greater than inhibition of butyrylcholinesterase.

Galantamine is also an allosteric modulator of nicotinic cholinergic receptors, a property that has been demonstrated in human nicotinic receptors expressed in cell lines [21]. Tacrine, donepezil, rivastigmine and metrifonate appear to be inactive in this model over a broad concentration range [21]. Nicotinic modulation is probably related to the chemical structure of galantamine and independent of its cholinesterase inhibition. It has been suggested that this may give the drug a different profile of clinical activity although this has to be confirmed.

Pharmacokinetics

The bioavailability of galantamine after oral administration is 85% with a plasma elimination half-life of about 6 h. It produces four metabolites, one of which is more active as an acetylcholinesterase inhibitor than galantamine itself [1]. Fifty per cent of galantamine is eliminated in urine, half as the metabolites and half unchanged. It does not bind significantly to plasma proteins.

Clinical evidence

Efficacy

The galantamine clinical trial programme has already included over 2000 patients in double-blind trials. Relative to placebo-treated patients, patients treated with galantamine have shown statistically significant improvements in both psychometric scales (ADAS-Cog) and clinician's interview-based assessments (CIBIC-Plus). For example, results have been presented [22] from an international study involving 653 patients with mild to moderate AD (215 on placebo, 220 on galantamine 24 mg/day, and 218 on galantamine 32 mg/day). Patients treated with galantamine over 6 months improved 1.7 points on average in comparison with a 2.4-point average deterioration in those receiving placebo. The majority of patients receiving galantamine 24 and 32 mg/day were also maintained or improved during the trial as assessed by the CIBIC-Plus. Very similar results were obtained with a pivotal US double-blind study involving 423 patients receiving galantamine twice daily for 6 months and 213 taking placebo.

Patients treated with galantamine for one year maintained their memory and cognitive function above baseline [23]. Those patients who had received placebo during the first six months of the international trial were transferred to galantamine 12 mg bd for the second 6-months. Their change in cognitive function did not reach that of the group receiving galantamine for 12 months continuously and the difference in outcomes between the two groups was significant ($p \leq 0.05$).

Other data suggest that after 6 months, by comparison with placebo, galantamine can reduce the time carers spend supervising patients by up to two hours a day [24].

Adverse events

The adverse event profile is similar to other cholinesterase inhibitors with nausea, vomiting and other gastrointestinal side-effects occurring at approximately two to four times the placebo rate but usually transient and subsiding within about a week.

Practical use

Indications

Mild to moderate AD.

Dosage and administration

Galantamine dosage has been expressed in different ways and this is potentially confusing especially when reviewing older published data. In some early studies, the dose of galantamine is expressed as galantamine hydrobromide (and requires a conversion factor of 0.8). All subsequent and current studies express the dose as galantamine itself. A dosage of 12 mg twice daily is likely to be the usual dose.

Place of galantamine in the management of Alzheimer's disease

At present there are no formal comparisons between different cholinesterase inhibitors. Anecdotally it seems that galantamine may potentially show greater efficacy but possibly with a higher level of side-effects that may be reduced by a slower dose escalation over 8 weeks [25].

Availability

A different formulation of the drug is already approved for treating AD in Austria (it is an old compound marketed previously there by Waldheim). The current formulation of galantamine is being codeveloped by Shire and Janssen-Cilag. It was recently approved in Sweden and is now being considered for approval as part of the European Union Mutual Recognition Procedure. Submissions have also been made in other countries, including the USA, Canada, New Zealand, Poland, Norway and Switzerland.

Metrifonate (Bayer)

Pharmacology

Mode of action

Metrifonate is an old treatment for schistosomiasis [26]. It is a pro-drug that is converted non-enzymatically to the potent cholinesterase inhibitor dichlorvos. It is a physiologically irreversible cholinesterase inhibitor inhibiting both acetylcholinesterase and butyrylcholinesterase.

Erythrocyte acetylcholinesterase activity was inhibited by 62 and 72% at steady state using a low- or high-dosage regimen, respectively. Dosing with metrifonate has usually involved a loading dose (2 mg/kg) followed by a maintenance dose (most effective 0.65 mg/kg/day).

Pharmacokinetics

The drug is absorbed rapidly after oral administration. Metrifonate and dichlorvos both have short plasma half-lives of around 2 h but the effects on the cholinesterase enzymes last for many days. Metrifonate undergoes little protein binding (< 15%).

Clinical evidence

Efficacy

Metrifonate has been studied in more than 2000 patients with mild to moderate AD. In a 26-week study of 408 patients [27], 135 patients received placebo and 273 metrifonate 100–180 mg loading dose for 2 weeks followed by 30–60 mg maintenance dose according to body weight. There was a significant improvement not only in cognitive function (2.86 points difference on the ADAS-Cog) and global assessment (0.28 points improvement on the CIBIC-Plus) but also in behaviour (with a change in the mean Neuropsychiatric Inventory (NPI) [see p. 33] total score). This is probably the first prospective double-blind study to show that a cholinesterase inhibitor can improve behavioural function and the first to show concurrent cognitive, global and behavioural benefit (although many earlier studies with metrifonate and other drugs would not have included behavioural instruments like the NPI).

In the MALT (Metrifonate Alzheimer Trial) [28], 605 patients took part in a 26-week trial receiving placebo, low dose (40 or 50 mg/day according to body weight) or high dose (60 or 80 mg), the latter two doses preceded by a 2-week loading dose period. Four clinical domains were assessed: cognition (using the ADAS-Cog and the MMSE), instrumental and basic ADL (using the Disability Assessment for Dementia [DAD]), behavioural and psychiatric disturbances ADL (using the ADAS-Noncog and the NPI) and global functioning and severity (using the CIBIC-Plus and the GDS). Significant differences were again demonstrated between metrifonate (high dose) and placebo for the four domains assessed, with a lesser degree of improvement for the lower dose.

Adverse events

The most common adverse events are dose-dependent cholinergic problems, typically gastrointestinal effects such as nausea, vomiting and diarrhoea, weakness and leg cramps. Although the adverse effects are generally mild, the withdrawal rate because of adverse events was three times greater for metrifonate (12%) than for placebo (4%) in one study [27]. Lower rates were found in the MALT study with 8% withdrawing because of adverse events on 60/80 mg drug daily in comparison to 6% on placebo [28].

Practical use

Indication

Mild to moderate AD.

Dosage and administration

The dose would originally have probably been 60–80 mg once daily, according to the weight of the patient. If metrifonate is developed further, it appears that lower doses will be used.

Place of metrifonate in the management of Alzheimer's disease

Although metrifonate has clearly demonstrated efficacy, trials were halted in 1998 because of concerns about severe muscle weakness seen in some trials in the USA. Full information about this is still not available although it is known from previous use of the drug that very high doses may cause neurotoxicity and polyneuropathy [26].

Availability

Not available. In 1998 the European licensing application was withdrawn and further information requested by the US FDA. The manufacturers have suggested that they still hope to register the drug but probably only at the lower doses tested.

Other cholinesterase inhibitors

Physostigmine was the earliest member of this group to be studied but, although effective, it has a very short half-life and is poorly tolerated. A twice-daily controlled-release version (Synapton) has been developed in the USA and data are apparently available on more than 2000 patients, some of whom have been on the drug for more than 6 years. Results of a 24-week double-blind placebo-controlled study in 475 patients with mild to moderate AD show similar efficacy to other cholinesterase inhibitors [29]. There was a 2.9-point ADAS-Cog difference between physostigmine and placebo and a significant improvement on the CIBIC-Plus. However, there was a high drop-out rate in the drug-treated group due to gastrointestinal side-effects. By comparison with the latest cholinesterase inhibitors physostigmine appears to have an unacceptable risk–benefit profile and is unlikely to be approved or marketed for AD.

Heptylphysostigmine (also called eptastigmine) is a long-acting orally active lipophilic derivative of physostigmine that was under development and appeared to show efficacy. In early 1999 its development was stopped apparently because of haematological adverse events including aplastic anaemias.

Huperzine A is an alkaloid derived from a traditional Chinese herbal remedy which is apparently still under development in the USA for AD. Development of velnacrine (Mentane) and quilostigmine (NXX-066) has been stopped.

Cholinergic agonists

Muscarinic agonists

Pharmacology

Cholinergic receptors are divided into two main types, muscarinic and nicotinic. There are pharmacologically distinct presynaptic and post-synaptic muscarinic receptors in the brain. In AD, it is the presynaptic neurone that is primarily affected. It might seem logical therefore to expect greater efficacy from muscarinic agonists that stimulate the postsynaptic (M1) receptor than from cholinesterase inhibitors that rely on the presence of the presynaptic production of acetylcholine.

Clinical evidence

Several muscarinic agonists have been studied in clinical trials. These include xanomeline, milameline, sabcomeline (Memric), SR46559 and alvameline, all of which have been dropped from further development.

Results with sabcomeline were typical for these compounds. The dose–response curve appeared shallow and the effects on cognitive function were inadequate at doses that were well tolerated. However, some benefit was seen on behavioural disturbance, a secondary endpoint, and this is being investigated further. Talsaclidine is the only remaining muscarinic agonist still under development for improvement of cognition in AD.

Although results with talsaclidine are awaited with interest, unfortunately it seems unlikely that a muscarinic agonist can be developed where adequate cognitive improvement is obtained with acceptable tolerability. However, such compounds may prove useful for behavioural disturbance in dementia.

Nicotinic agonists

Pharmacology

Nicotinic cholinergic receptors occur in significant numbers in the brain and are important in learning and memory. There is a reduction in nicotinic receptors in the cortex in AD that correlates with the severity of the symptoms.

Studies of nicotine in animals and humans have shown that nicotinic antagonists like mecamylamine impair memory and cognitive performance. On the other hand, nicotine itself can facilitate memory and attention in learning paradigms in animals and also in humans.

Cigarette smoking increases the number of brain nicotinic receptors. There has been interest in reports that smokers may be protected against AD. The relationship between smoking, vascular disease, apolipoprotein E4 and AD is complex but more recent data suggest that smokers have double the risk for dementia and AD [30].

Clinical evidence

Nicotine is reported to improve attention and information processing in AD patients and there have been small studies looking at the use of nicotine patches [31].

Further research is needed to confirm whether nicotine or nicotinic agonists such as ABT-418 are effective and of use in AD or other dementias. They are also likely to have marked vascular effects so any benefit must be balanced by an acceptable side-effect profile.

Another approach that has attracted attention recently is the development of compounds that modulate the activity of nicotinic receptors. These include codeine, physostigmine and galantamine. As previously mentioned (see p. 49) galantamine is an acetylcholin-esterase inhibitor and it is not clear whether this additional activity of the drug will translate into a real clinical difference between it and some of the other cholinesterase inhibitors.

This is an area that is continuing to develop, and new nicotinic agonists and nicotinic receptor modulators may be developed in the future. Direct stimulation by nicotinic agonists may induce desensitization of nicotinic receptors reducing the efficacy of such compounds in the longer term. Receptors modulation may therefore be the better approach because it should avoid this [32].

Acetyl-L-carnitine (Alcar; Sigma-Tau/Roche)

Mechanism of action

This compound is an esterified form of L-carnitine that crosses the blood–brain barrier. Historically it was considered to be a cholinergic agent either as a partial cholinergic agonist or because it can be converted to acetylcholine in the brain. It may act on other neurotransmitters and may be neuroprotective [33] with antioxidant properties, membrane stabilization effects and preservation of mitochondrial function.

Clinical efficacy

The drug has been under study for dementia for a number of years and several studies have been published. Doses have ranged from 300 to 3000 mg/day. Placebo-controlled studies suggest that the drug does have beneficial effects, for example on short-term memory and on deterioration in cognitive function. A more recent larger double-blind study suggests that the drug may slow the progression of AD in younger subjects [34].

Further large-scale studies are needed if this drug is to be licensed.

Indirect enhancement of cholinergic activity

Nerve growth factors

Pharmacology

Nerve growth factors (NGFs) are a group of naturally occurring compounds that are important in the development and maintenance of the vertebrate nervous system. NGF itself has its effects on central cholinergic neurones. So far, there is no direct evidence that a decline in NGF-related mechanisms is involved in AD pathogenesis. However, NGF might be effective in restoring a dysfunctional cholinergic system and there is evidence that many cholinergic basal forebrain neurones survive. Intracerebroventricular NGF infusions can modify damage to these neurones in animal models.

Clinical evidence

NGF has been infused into the lateral ventricles of three patients with AD for up to 3 months [35]. Whilst there was an increase in nicotine binding sites, a clear cognitive benefit could not be demonstrated. The infusions were associated with a dull, constant back pain and weight loss.

Place of nerve growth factor in the management of Alzheimer's disease

There are two main problems with this approach. Firstly, it will be difficult to ensure specificity of action of NGFs to the particular cholinergic neurones. Secondly, the NGFs do not pass the blood–brain barrier, hence the need for intraventricular infusions. It may be possible to develop forms of NGF or synthetic analogues that are orally active, and research is also examining the use of other routes such as intranasal delivery.

Glutamate modulators

Pharmacology

Glutamate, the most prevalent excitatory neurotransmitter in the brain, may also be important in the pathogenesis of dementia. Its role in dementias such as Alzheimer's disease is complex; there are theoretical reasons to support therapies that either might enhance glutamatergic hypoactivity or inhibit excessive glutamate activity.

It is the main fast excitatory neurotransmitter in the cerebral cortex and hippocampus and the neurotransmitter of the neocortical pyramidal cells, the neurones that are selectively lost in Alzheimer's disease [36].

Glutamate antagonists cause memory and learning deficits in animals and there is a correlation between loss of pyramidal cells and the severity of cognitive deficit.

There are a number of excitatory amino acid receptors. One of these, the NMDA (N-Methyl-D-aspartate) receptor, is of particular interest because of its capability for long-term potentiation which is probably a prerequisite for memory formation.

In contrast to glutamate hypoactivity in dementia, glutamate may also have an important role because of its action as an excitotoxin causing neuronal death when excessive levels are chronically released.

In animal models, neurodegeneration occurs on exposure to high concentrations of excitatory amino acids (EAA). This led to a glutamatergic hypothesis of dementia suggesting that excess activation may underlie disorders including Huntington's disease and AD. EAA toxicity may also be important in ischaemic damage such as stroke when glutamate release is greatly increased. Interestingly β-amyloid may enhance EAA toxicity in neurone cultures by enhancing calcium influx.

Memantine (Akatinol; Merz)

Mechanism of action

Memantine was originally marketed as an antispasticity agent. It acts as an uncompetitive antagonist at the NMDA receptor, blocking glutamate-gated receptor channels, allowing the physiological activation of the receptors whilst blocking their pathological activation. Memantine acts like magnesium, blocking NMDA receptor channels in the resting state whilst leaving the channel on physiological activation during memory formation. In contrast to magnesium, it does not leave the channel under pathological activation. In animal models, it provides neuroprotection against the excitotoxic activation of glutamate receptors, whilst preserving or even restoring their physiological activation [36].

Clinical evidence

Efficacy

Memantine has been evaluated in AD and VaD in short-term (4–6 weeks), placebo-controlled clinical trials involving more than 500 patients with mild to moderate dementia. The usual daily dose ranged from 20 to 30 mg, and significant improvements in cognitive disturbance, drive and motor functions were observed.

There are also data from a recent study [36] in patients with severe dementia using 10 mg memantine per day that suggested clinically relevant and significant improvement in functioning, care dependence and behavioural symptoms over a period of 12 weeks.

Adverse events

The most frequent adverse events have been vertigo, restlessness, hyperexcitation, fatigue, diarrhoea and gastric pain, but there were no major differences in frequency between the drug and placebo.

Indications

Memantine is currently being evaluated in AD (including severe AD), VaD and in the USA for AIDS-related dementia.

Availability

The drug is already available in Germany, Luxemburg and Portugal for the treatment of spasticity and/or dementia.

Place of memantine in the management of Alzheimer's disease and dementia

Memantine is one of the few drugs so far to have been evaluated in more severe dementia. Early trials with the compound used methodology that would not now be acceptable. Several large-scale trials in mild to moderate dementia using current methodology are now complete and the results from these are awaited with interest. If the results are positive, the data will be used to submit applications to register the drug worldwide for use in dementia.

Glial cell modulators

Propentofylline (Aventis Pharma)

Pharmacology

Propentofylline (HWA 285) is a novel xanthine derivative that has been developed for AD and VaD. Various pharmacological properties support its potential as a neuroprotective agent, although it is usually described as a glial cell modulator.

- It enhances extracellular adenosine levels by inhibiting its reuptake.
- It is a phosphodiesterase inhibitor.
- It modulates the activation of microglial cells suppressing their neurotoxic effects.
- It restores impaired astrocyte function by stimulating synthesis/release of NGF.

These actions suggest that propentofylline might have a different clinical profile in comparison to neurotransmitter-based strategies. It might cause less immediate symptomatic improvement but have a greater impact on stabilizing disease progression in the longer term.

Pharmacokinetics

Few published data are available [37]. However, it is known that the oral absorption of the drug is significantly affected by the presence of food in the stomach for up to 4 h after intake of the meal.

Clinical evidence

Efficacy

A review of four phase III trials has been published [38]. The studies involved 901 patients with mild to moderate AD (MMSE 15–25) and 359 patients with mild to moderate VaD. The double-blind, placebo-controlled, randomized studies ranged in duration from 6 months to 56 weeks.

Propentofylline showed consistent improvements over placebo for both AD and VaD. As usual, drug efficacy was assessed in the three domains of cognitive performance, global function and ADL. In AD there were statistically significant effects on cognition with corresponding statistically significant improvement in global function and to some extent in ADL. Similar effects were seen in VaD for cognitive and global function.

At the end of the study there was no significant deterioration of patients after discontinuing treatment for 8 weeks [38] in contrast with data for cholinergic drugs [7]. This difference is compatible with the concept that the drug may have an effect on the disease process rather than just acting symptomatically.

Adverse events

The most frequent adverse events possibly related to propentofylline are nausea, dizziness, headache, gastrointestinal disturbances and vasodilatation [37,38]. In general the drug appears to be well tolerated.

Practical use

Indications

Propentofylline is intended for use in AD and VaD.

Dosage and administration

The dose that has been studied is 300 mg three times daily with few available data at other doses. The drug must be taken on an empty stomach at least 1 h before food.

Availability

Propentofylline as Hextol has actually been available in Japan for 'cerebral metabolism and related disorders'. The efficacy of compounds for this indication has been reviewed and the drug delisted along with several other compounds.

In October 1998 the European CPMP voted not to recommend approval of propentofylline for the treatment of AD or VaD, and an appeal against the decision for AD was rejected in March 1999. The data, although positive, were not sufficient to recommend approval. Another pivotal phase III study in AD was scheduled to take place in the USA before further licensing applications. However, in March 2000, Aventis Pharma discontinued development of the drug. This followed a review of their overall portfolio and because of results from the more recent 72-week Propentofylline Long-term Use Study (PLUS) where no treatment differences were seen between the drug and placebo.

Place of propentofylline in the management of Alzheimer's disease and vascular dementia

Although potentially valuable, because of its different activity profile, proving relevant efficacy and satisfying regulatory authorities has been difficult for several reasons. Even if effective, there may be little immediate benefit if it stabilizes or delays the disease process. Also, there is still uncertainty about the reliability of its absorption and its interaction with food. This may limit its usefulness because of practical difficulties with three times daily dosing and ensuring that patients take it well away from food.

Antioxidants and monoamine oxidase inhibitors

Monoamine oxidase B inhibitors

Mechanism of action

Monoamine oxidase B (MAO-B) activity in platelets and brain tissue is increased in AD and this may be pathological. As a result, there has been interest in whether MAO-B inhibitors, by increasing catecholamine levels, can enhance cognitive function. Another possibility is that drugs such as selegiline, a selective MAO-B inhibitor at low doses (10 mg/day), act as antioxidants when inhibiting oxidative deamination thereby reducing neuronal damage. This action will be considered further in the next section on antioxidants.

Clinical evidence

Selegiline (L-deprenyl)

In 1996, a review evaluated the effects of selegiline on cognitive and behavioural symptoms in AD [39]. Seventeen studies assessing cognition and eight assessing behaviour were considered. All non-double-blind studies gave positive results as did eight of the 11 double-blind, placebo-controlled studies assessing cognition and two of the five assessing behavioural improvement.

The review did not insist on strict inclusion criteria so that poorly designed studies were still assessed. Overall, the trials do suggest that selegiline may be useful in treating behavioural and cognitive symptoms. The authors correctly state that selegiline's role in AD needs clarifying with larger well-controlled and longer-term clinical trials.

A more recent 6-month study of selegiline (10 mg daily) or placebo did not show any detectable benefit on general behaviour, neuropsychiatric symptoms or cognitive function in AD [40].

Milacemide and lazabemide

Two other MAO-B inhibitors investigated for use in AD are milacemide and lazabemide. Milacemide was tested as a potential cognitive enhancer but did not demonstrate adequate efficacy and development was halted. Lazabemide, another reversible MAO-B inhibitor, appeared promising but development was recently stopped because of concerns about hepatic toxicity.

Vitamin E (alpha-tocopherol) and selegiline

Mechanism of action

Ageing is associated with free radical damage and is the main risk factor for AD. There is also evidence of increased lipid peroxidation in the AD brain. Free radicals appear to initiate and maintain the cascade of events that leads to neurodegeneration. Antioxidants have the potential to reduce neuronal damage and thus slow the progression of AD.

Selegiline may act as an antioxidant and also increases levels of catecholamines; vitamin E is a lipid-soluble vitamin which traps oxygen free radicals, and interrupts the chain reaction that damages cells.

Clinical evidence

In a recent randomized, controlled trial [41], 341 patients with moderately severe AD received selegiline (5 mg b.d.), vitamin E (1000 IU b.d.), both selegiline and vitamin E, or placebo for 2 years. The primary outcomes were the time to occurrence of death or institutionalization or loss of the ability to perform basic ADL or severe dementia. Although there are concerns about the appropriateness of the end-points and the validity of the statistical analysis, treatment with selegiline or vitamin E delayed the progression of the disease by 215–230 days. Further efficacy studies will be awaited with interest particularly in patients with mild cognitive impairment or early dementia.

Place of antioxidants in the treatment of Alzheimer's disease

Of the two treatments, vitamin E is the more innocuous, although at high doses it may augment coagulation defects in patients with vitamin K deficiency. It seems reasonable to consider vitamin E in patients with mild to moderate AD. Although the data are for higher doses (2000 IU/day), the American Psychiatric Association [42] suggest that conventional doses (200–800 IU/day) are used.

Selegiline is an alternative but vitamin E is cheaper, better tolerated and with less potential for drug interactions. On the other hand, selegiline may actually improve cognition and behaviour as well as delay functional decline. It might be considered therefore for those who cannot take cholinesterase inhibitors [42].

Ginkgo biloba

Extracts from the leaves of the *Ginkgo biloba* (maidenhair) tree have been widely used in China for thousands of years for various conditions. More recently there has been widespread interest in its use as a cognitive enhancer.

Pharmacology

Mode of action

Several actions have been described. The effects may be caused by single ingredients or by the combined action of the many agents in the extracts. These include flavonoids, terpenoids (including several ginkgolides that are unique to the ginkgo tree) and organic acids.

The mechanisms include: effects on the vasoregulatory activity of arteries, capillaries and veins increasing blood flow; antagonism of platelet-activating factor; metabolic changes, for example on neurone metabolism increasing tolerance to anoxia; and prevention of membrane damage caused by free radicals. In dementia, the most important action may be the ability of the constituents, perhaps working synergistically, to mop up free radicals preventing excessive lipid peroxidation and nerve cell injury.

Pharmacokinetics

It is difficult to assess the pharmacokinetics of ginkgo extracts because of the multiple active ingredients. There are very few satisfactory published data.

Clinical evidence

Efficacy

Although most studies have been of poor quality, a double-blind placebo-controlled trial in dementia was carried out in the USA using current methods for entry and assessment [43]. The study included 327 patients with AD or multi-infarct dementia, 309 of whom were included in the intent-to-treat analysis. There was a high withdrawal rate with only 50% of ginkgo patients completing 52 weeks compared with 38% for placebo. There was no significant change in the ADAS-Cog score at 52 weeks for the ginkgo group whereas the placebo group had deteriorated by a mean of 1.5 points (much less than would normally be expected). Patients on placebo were worse on a daily living and social behaviour scale whereas there was a continuing small improvement on the active drug. The between-group differences for both measures were highly significant but not for a clinician's global measure of change.

Ginkgo stabilized and, in some cases, improved the cognitive performance and social function of demented patients for 6–12 months. The changes were modest but were objectively measured by the ADAS-Cog and also recognized by the carers as a significant change in a caregiver-rating scale.

The results allow calculation of the NNT to obtain a 4-point ADAS-Cog improvement (4 points represent the average deterioration that would be expected over a 6-month period in untreated subjects) or for an improvement in daily living and social behaviour to be noticed by the patient's family. For ADAS-Cog scores, the NNT was 7.9 (95% CI 4.2–67) for all dementia patients and 6.3 (3.5–32) for AD patients. For a patient's family to notice an improvement in daily living and social behaviour about 7 patients with dementia or 5.3 patients with AD need to be treated for 1 year but the confidence intervals are again wide (3.3–97 for dementia, 2.9–28 for AD) [43a].

In 1998 a formal review [44] of more than 50 articles, mostly in the French and German literature, only found four that could be used in a meta-analysis. Most were rejected because there was no clear diagnosis of dementia or AD. In total there were 212 subjects in each of the placebo and ginkgo groups. There appeared to be a small but positive effect of 3–6-months' treatment with 120–240 mg of *Ginkgo biloba* extract on objective measures of cognitive function in AD (equivalent to a 3% difference in the ADAS-Cog subtest). There was also some preliminary evidence in two of the four studies for efficacy in VaD. It was difficult to be clear whether there were effects on non-cognitive behavioural and functional measures or clinician's global ratings.

Adverse events

No serious drug-related side-effects have been noted. Rarely, mild gastrointestinal complaints, headache and allergic skin reactions have been reported as have two reports of bleeding complications that may be linked to antagonism of platelet-activating factor. It would seem prudent to be cautious in patients taking anticoagulants, antiplatelet agents or with a bleeding diathesis [44].

Practical use

Indications

Ginkgo extracts have been used for a variety of indications such as cerebral insufficiency where the exact clinical diagnosis is unclear. In the more recent double-blind study [43], patients were included with mild to moderately severe (MMSE score 9–26) AD or multi-infarct dementia.

Dosage and administration

Numerous preparations of ginkgo are available and their composition, purity and standardization may vary. Controlled trials have been limited to four preparations: Tebonin, Tanakan, rökan and Kaveri. The first three are different names for the same extract EGb761 and use standardized amounts of ginkgo-flavone glycosides (24%) and terpenoids (6%). Kaveri is also called LI370 and is also standardized on the same ingredients with similar doses.

The usual dose range is 120–240 mg.

Availability

It is available in many European countries as an over-the-counter product for the treatment of cerebral vascular insufficiency and tinnitus. Certain preparations are marketed for 'intellectual deficit' in France and for dementia in Germany. Ginkgo extracts are marketed by many different companies.

Place of ginkgo in the management of dementia

Ginkgo extracts are popular in Europe and there have been attempts to develop this for more widespread licensing. One problem is identifying the active ingredient(s) and without this regulatory approval in many countries is unlikely. There is evidence of some efficacy with regard to cognition. Further research is needed to determine if there are functional improvements. Information on dosage is still unclear.

Anti-inflammatory agents

Mechanism of action

Inflammatory mechanisms appear to be an important part of the AD process and may play a part in other dementias. It seems likely that the brain generates an inflammatory response to the underlying disease process, inflammation then contributing to the continuing neurodegenerative process.

Many laboratories have confirmed the potential involvement of inflammatory and immune mechanisms. Acute-phase proteins, particularly α_1-antichymotrypsin, are elevated in the serum and also deposited in neuritic plaques; activated microglial cells that stain for inflammatory cytokines are associated with neuritic but not diffuse plaques, and may be involved in the conversion of diffuse plaques to neuritic plaques; complement components are present around dystrophic neurites and neurofibrillary tangles; and the complement component C1q is associated with amyloid deposits in the AD brain. Lysosomal activity may also be important in the amyloidogenic breakdown of amyloid precursor protein.

Clinical evidence

Epidemiological evidence

More than 20 epidemiological studies support the possibility that anti-inflammatory drugs delay the onset and/or progression of AD. Most are cross-sectional or case–control studies and potentially liable to under-reporting from patients with AD or their families. Nevertheless, a meta-analysis in 1996 reviewing 17 epidemiological studies [45] suggested that anti-inflammatory treatment might decrease the risk of developing AD by as much as 50%.

In a prospective study [46], part of the Baltimore Longitudinal Study of Ageing, the relative risk (RR) for AD decreased with increasing duration of non-steroidal anti-inflammatory drug (NSAID) use. In those with 2 or more years of reported NSAID use, the RR was 0.40 (95% CI: 0.19–0.84) compared with 0.65 (95% CI: 0.33–1.29) for those with less than 2 years use. The effect of aspirin was less convincing but may be confounded by people taking low-dose aspirin (sufficient to affect platelet aggregation) rather than anti-inflammatory doses. As would be expected, no benefit was found for taking paracetamol which is not an anti-inflammatory drug.

Efficacy

There are only a limited number of published prospective double-blind studies examining the potential of anti-inflammatory drugs. In a 6-month study using indomethacin at doses of 100–150 mg/day [47], indomethacin-treated patients improved slightly on a battery of cognitive tests whereas placebo-treated patients declined; the differences were statistically significant.

A small open-label pilot study with prednisone 10 or 20 mg did not show significant changes in cognition or behaviour but at 20 mg some acute-phase serum proteins were reduced [48].

Adverse events

There are undoubtedly risks of unpleasant and potentially serious adverse effects from anti-inflammatory medication and these are more common in elderly people. For example, in the 6-month indomethacin efficacy study mentioned above, a quarter of the indomethacin group could not tolerate the treatment (because of gastrointestinal problems or headaches) and were withdrawn.

Place of anti-inflammatory agents in the management of dementia

There does seem to be a potentially important benefit from taking regular anti-inflammatory medication. In view of their toxicity, they cannot be recommended for general use in dementia until further controlled trials with adequate numbers of subjects have been conducted.

A number of larger prospective double-blind studies are apparently now in progress using a range of compounds. These include NSAIDs, corticosteroids, hydroxychloroquine and colchicine. Colchicine inhibits lysosomal activity (as does hydroxychloroquine) and is already used in treating other amyloidoses.

There is considerable interest in the possible advantages of NSAIDs that are more selective for cyclooxygenase-2 (COX-2) thereby decreasing inflammation while preserving gastric function. These include nabumetone (Relifex), etodolac (Lodine) and meloxicam (Mobic). Two highly selective COX-2 inhibitors, celecoxib and rofecoxib, are just becoming available on prescription in several countries and are already being assessed for potential efficacy in AD.

Oestrogens

Several studies have suggested that oestrogen replacement therapy in postmenopausal women may improve cognitive function and be associated with a delay in the onset of dementia and a reduction in the severity of cognitive decline.

Mechanism of action

Oestrogens may affect cognitive function through a number of possible mechanisms: prevention of neuronal atrophy (for example in the hippocampus); acting as a cofactor in the effects of NGFs; promotion of cholinergic and serotonergic activity in specific brain regions; prevention of cerebral ischaemia; and through favourable alterations in lipoproteins [49].

Clinical evidence

There has been a meta-analysis of 10 observational studies (published between 1984 and 1997) that measured the effect of postmenopausal oestrogen use [49]. Whilst there appeared to be a decreased risk of developing dementia, the findings were heterogeneous and there were potential methodological problems. For example, women who choose to take oestrogens are reported to be better educated and healthier than non-users, differences that may in any case reduce the risk of AD [49].

Four trials of oestrogen therapy involving 58 women with AD were also reviewed. Although results were primarily positive, the studies were mainly uncontrolled, unblinded and non-randomized.

Place of oestrogens in the management of dementia and Alzheimer's disease

In view of the risks of therapy, the authors of the above review do not recommend oestrogen for the prevention or treatment of AD or other dementias until adequate trials have been completed. However, postmenopausal women considering the overall risks and benefits of oestrogen replacement therapy may want to consider this preliminary evidence [42].

Older compounds still sometimes used

There are a number of older drugs that are still important in some countries. These include co-dergocrine mesylate (Hydergine), naftidrofuryl oxalate (Praxilene), piracetam and other related so-called nootropic agents.

Co-dergocrine mesylate (Hydergine)

Hydergine is the brand name for a particular combination of four dihydro derivatives of ergotoxine, referred to as co-dergocrine mesylate, which has been available since 1949. It has been used for peripheral vascular disease, angina, hypertension and tinnitus. It is still widely used but almost exclusively for treating people with dementia or age-related cognitive symptoms. It is approved in the USA for 'idiopathic decline in mental capacity' and in the UK 'as an adjunct in the management of elderly patients with mild to moderate dementia'. The drug has been advocated as a so-called 'smart drug' for use by young and older normal adults to increase mental ability.

There has always been uncertainty surrounding its efficacy. This is more difficult because most trials were carried out some years ago when diagnostic criteria were non-specific and the trial methodology was fairly crude. Several detailed reviews have been published over the years, most recently a systematic Cochrane review [50]. All agree that there are significant effects favouring co-dergocrine, for example in helping some patients with their ADL, their symptoms and their self-care. Greater effect sizes on global ratings were associated with younger age and possibly higher dose (including doses above the US recommended upper limit of 3 mg/day). The drug was well tolerated. Overall, the improvements appear small and the reviewers remain uncertain about co-dergocrine's efficacy. It may be having a more general effect on mood rather than a specifically antidementia effect.

Piracetam and other nootropic agents

Nootropic agents were named because of their apparent ability to improve integrative brain mechanisms associated with mental performance. Such agents should enhance learning and memory and the general resistance of the brain to external physical and chemical injuries (e.g. as a result of hypoxia or barbiturate poisoning); they are also characterized by none of the usual psychological and general cardiovascular pharmacological activities. Nootropics do not have a well-defined mechanism of action. The term has been mainly applied to piracetam and piracetam-like compounds (e.g. pramiracetam, aniracetam and oxiracetam).

Piracetam (2-oxo-1-pyrrolidine acetamide) was the first nootropic and is a cyclic derivative of γ-aminobutyric acid (GABA) which can cross the blood–brain barrier and concentrates in the cortex. The benefits of piracetam in patients with AD, VaD and unspecified dementia are still controversial. Such compounds have never been approved in Anglo-Saxon countries because of this equivocal efficacy; however, piracetam is widely used for cognitive impairment and dementia in several European countries. A recent systematic review [51] concluded that the published evidence available does not support piracetam's use in the treatment of dementia or cognitive impairment because effects were found only on global impression of change but not on more specific measures.

Naftidrofuryl oxalate (Praxilene)

Naftidrofuryl oxalate, an acid ester of diethylaminoethanol, is another compound that has been available for many years. In the UK it is licensed for peripheral and cerebral vascular disorders, specifically cerebral insufficiency and cerebral atherosclerosis, particularly where these manifest themselves as mental deterioration and confusion in the elderly. Its pharmacological actions remain poorly understood. Naftidrofuryl's clinical effects are attributed to actions on cellular metabolism increasing adenosine triphosphate stores and regional blood flow. As with co-dergocrine, most trials were carried out some years ago when diagnostic criteria were non-specific and trial methodology was still crude. Although several short-term studies have shown modest effects, there has been no definitive improvement in cognition, nor is it clear whether there are sustained benefits. It seems unlikely that naftidrofuryl would qualify as an effective antidementia therapy according to modern regulatory and clinical expectations.

Vascular dementia

Aspirin

For patients with a diagnosis of VaD there is evidence that aspirin is widely prescribed. In a study completed by UK geriatricians and psychiatrists [52], more than 80% of patients with cognitive impairment and vascular risk factors were prescribed aspirin. In a recent systematic review [52] 11 publications were identified as potentially relevant but only one randomized controlled trial of aspirin in VaD was identified. Data for analysis were available for 70 patients but only with regard to cognition. There was a change in cognitive outcome that was towards being in favour of aspirin treatment. No information is available with regard to other outcomes such as behaviour, quality of life and effects on time to institutionalization.

So many patients with dementia are given low doses of aspirin for one reason or another that it may prove difficult to carry out the appropriate studies to clarify its efficacy or otherwise.

Cholinesterase inhibitors

Recent animal and human data suggest that there are similar cholinergic deficits to those in AD in vascular lesions in the brain of animals and VaD patients. There are also anecdotal reports that cholinesterase inhibitors improve cognitive deficits associated with stroke. At present, formal studies are in progress to evaluate the efficacy of cholinesterase inhibitors in VaD.

Dementia with Lewy bodies

Cholinesterase inhibitors

Analysis of clinical trials with cholinesterase inhibitors in AD confirm that only a subgroup of patients respond to the treatment. In most studies, the criteria used for diagnosing AD mean that some 10–20% of patients may have an alternative explanation for their dementia [53]. In addition, there is considerable heterogeneity in AD and at post mortem cortical Lewy bodies may be found in a significant number of cases either together with, or independently of, AD changes. The profound cholinergic deficit in dementia with Lewy bodies (DLB) (see Chapter 1, p. 7) gives theoretical support for cholinesterase inhibitors being as, or even more, effective in this condition than in AD.

There has been some clinical support for this with both tacrine and donepezil. For example, in a study with tacrine, people with DLB improved more frequently than those with AD [54]. The response was qualitatively different with a greater improvement in attention whereas in AD there was a greater improvement in conceptualization. Case studies also support an effect on psychotic symptoms as well as on cognition and parkinsonism. Preliminary data are emerging from a formal prospective study with rivastigmine that again suggests that cholinesterase inhibitors may have a useful role in the treatment of DLB.

Disease-modifying strategies

The overlap with AD pathology supports the evaluation of similar neuroprotective approaches in DLB. This would include anti-inflammatory and antioxidant medication, although selegiline is best avoided because it can precipitate hallucinations.

Avoidance of neuroleptic medication

The most important therapeutic action in DLB is to avoid the use of neuroleptic medication. These cause a sensitivity reaction in up to 50% of cases that can precipitate severe or irreversible parkinsonism as well as other manifestations and can be fatal. Although atypical neuroleptics are said to be better, they can also cause similar reactions.

References

1 Nordberg A, Svensson A-L. Cholinesterase inhibitors in the treatment of Alzheimer's disease: a comparison of tolerability and pharmacology. *Drug Safety* 1998; 19 (6): 465–80.

2 Wagstaff AJ, McTavish D. Tacrine: a review of its pharmacodynamic and pharmacokinetic properties, and therapeutic efficacy in Alzheimer's disease. *Drugs Aging* 1994; 4 (6): 510–40.

3 Arrieta JL, Artalejo FR. Methodology, results and quality of clinical trials of tacrine in the treatment of Alzheimer's disease: a systematic review of the literature. *Age Ageing* 1998; 27: 161–79.

4 Qizilbash N, Whitehead A, Higgins J *et al.* Cholinesterase inhibition for Alzheimer's disease: a meta-analysis of the tacrine trials. *JAMA* 1998; 280: 1777–82.

5 Cummings JL, Kaufer D. Neuropsychiatric aspects of Alzheimer's disease: the cholinergic hypothesis revisited. *Neurology* 1996; 47: 876–83.

6 Knopman D, Schneider L, Davis K *et al.* Long-term tacrine (Cognex) treatment: effects on nursing home placement and mortality. *Neurology* 1996; 47: 166–77.

7 Rogers SL, Farlow MR, Doody RS *et al.* A 24-week, double-blind, placebo-controlled trial of donepezil in patients with Alzheimer's disease. *Neurology* 1998; 50: 136–45.

8 Allen H. Anti-dementia drugs. *Int J Geriatr Psychiatry* 1999; 14: 239–43.

9 Rogers SL, Friedhoff LT. Long-term efficacy and safety of donepezil in the treatment of Alzheimer's disease: an interim analysis of the results of a US multicentre open label extension study. *Eur Neuropsychopharmacol* 1998; 8: 67–75.

10 Evans M, Ellis A, Watson D, Chowdhury T. Sustained cognitive improvement following treatment of Alzheimer's disease with donepezil. *Int J Geriatr Psychiatry* 2000; 15: 50–3.

11 Birks JS, Melzer D. Donepezil for mild and moderate Alzheimer's disease (Cochrane Review). In: *The Cochrane Library*, Issue 3. Oxford: Update Software, 1999.

12 Matthews HP, Jorbey J, Wilkinson DG, Rowden J. Donepezil in the treatment of Alzheimer's disease: results from the first 18 months of a study in clinical practice in the UK. *Eur Neuropsychopharmacol* 1999; 9 (Suppl. 5): S327.

13 Winblad B, Engedal K, Soininen H *et al.* Donepezil enhances global function, cognition and activities of daily living compared to placebo in a 1-year double-blind trial in patients with mild to moderate Alzheimer's disease. Abstract. *Ninth Congress of the International Psychogeriatric Association*, Vancouver, Canada, 1999.

14 Birks J, Iakovidou V, Tsolaki M. Rivastigmine for Alzheimer's disease (Cochrane Review). In: *The Cochrane Library*, Issue 3. Oxford: Update Software, 1999.

15 Schneider LS, Anand R, Farlow MR. Systematic review of the efficacy of rivastigmine for patients with Alzheimer's disease. *Int J Geriatr Psychopharmacol* 1998; 1: S26–S34.

16 Stein K. *Rivastigmine (Exelon) in the Treatment of Senile Dementia of the Alzheimer Type.* DEC Report no. 89. Bristol: NHS Executive South and West, 1998.

17 Spencer CM, Noble S. Rivastigmine: a review of its use in Alzheimer's disease. *Drugs Aging* 1998; 13 (5): 391–411.

18 Corey-Bloom J, Anand R, Veach J *et al.* A randomized trial evaluating the efficacy and safety of ENA 713 (rivastigmine tartrate), a new acetylcholinesterase inhibitor, in patients with mild to moderately severe Alzheimer's disease. *Int J Geriatr Psychopharmacol* 1998; 1: 55–65.

19 Rosler M, Anand R, Cicin-Sain A *et al.* Efficacy and safety of rivastigmine in patients with Alzheimer's disease: international, randomised controlled trial. *BMJ* 1999; 318: 633–40.

20 Anand R, Messina J, Hartman R, Graham S, Cicin-Sain A. Maximising functional ability: new data with cholinesterase inhibitors. Abstract. *Ninth Congress of the International Psychogeriatric Association*, Vancouver, Canada, 1999.

21 Maelicke A, Albuquerque EX. Allosteric modulation of nicotine acetyl choline receptors as treatment strategy for Alzheimer's disease. *Eur J Pharmacol* 2000 (in press).

22 Parys W, Pontecorvo MJ. Treatment of Alzheimer's disease with galantamine, a compound with a dual mode of action. Abstract, *6th International*

Conference on Alzheimer's Disease and Related Conditions, Amsterdam, Netherlands, 1998.

23 Parys W. Galantamine, a cognitive enhancer with nicotinic modulation: clinical benefits in Alzheimer's disease. Abstract, *4th Annual Congress of the European Federation of Neurological Societies*, Lisbon, Portugal, 1999.

24 Blesa R. Galantamine: therapeutic effects beyond cognition. Abstract, *4th Annual Congress of the European Federation of Neurological Societies*, Lisbon, Portugal, 1999.

25 Tariot P, Parys W, Kershaw P. The tolerability of galantamine in Alzheimer's disease: a 5-month placebo-controlled study with slow-dose escalation. *Sixth International Stockholm/Springfield Symposium*, Stockholm, Sweden, April 2000.

26 Lamb HM, Faulds D. Metrifonate. *Drugs Aging* 1997; 11: 490–6.

27 Morris JC, Cyrus PA, Orazem J *et al.* Metrifonate benefits cognitive, behavioral, and global function in patients with Alzheimer's disease. *Neurology* 1998; 50: 1222–30.

28 McKeith IG. The clinical trial protocol of the metrifonate in Alzheimer's trial (MALT). *Dement Geriatr Cogn Disord* 1998; 9 (Suppl. 2): 2–7.

29 Thal LJ, Ferguson JM, Mintzer J, Raskin A, Targum SD. A 24-week randomized trial of controlled-release physostigmine in patients with Alzheimer's disease. *Neurology* 1999; 52: 1146–52.

30 Ott A, Breteler MMB, van Harskamp F, Hofman A. Smoking increases the risk of dementia: the Rotterdam study. *Neurology* 1997; 48: A78.

31 White HK, Levin ED. Four-week nicotine skin patch treatment effects on cognitive performance in Alzheimer's disease. *Psychopharmacol* 1999; 143: 158–65.

32 Maelicke A, Albuquerque EX. New approach to drug therapy in Alzheimer's disease. *Drug Discovery Today* 1996; 1(2): 53–9.

33 Calvani M, Carta A, Caruso G, Benedetti N, Iannuccelli M. Action of acetyl-L-carnitine in neurodegeneration and Alzheimer's disease. *Ann N Y Acad Sci* 1992; 663: 483–6.

34 Brooks JO, Yesavage JA, Carta A, Bravi D. Acetyl-L-carnitine slows decline in younger patients with Alzheimer's disease. *Int Psychogeriatr* 1998; 10 (2): 193–203.

35 Eriksdotter JM, Nordberg A, Amberla K *et al.* Intracerebroventricular infusion of nerve growth factor in three patients with Alzheimer's disease. *Dement Geriatr Cogn Disord* 1998; 9 (5): 246–57.

36 Winblad B, Poritis N. Memantine in severe dementia: results of the M-BEST study (benefit and efficacy in severely demented patients during treatment with memantine). *Int J Geriatr Psychiatry* 1999; 14: 135–46.

37 Noble S, Wagstaff AJ. Propentofylline. *CNS Drugs* 1997; 8 (3): 257–66.

38 Rother M, Erkinjuntti T, Roessner M *et al.* Propentofylline in the treatment of Alzheimer's disease and vascular dementia: a review of phase III trials. *Dement Geriatr Cogn Disord* 1998; 9 (Suppl. 1): 36–43.

39 Tolbert SR, Fuller MA. Selegiline in treatment of behavioral and cognitive symptoms of Alzheimer's disease. *Ann Pharmacotherapy* 1996; 30: 1122–9.

40 Freedman M. L-Deprenyl in Alzheimer's disease: cognitive and behavioral effects. *Neurology* 1998; 50: 660–8.

41 Sano M, Ernesto MS, Thomas RG *et al.* A controlled trial of selegiline, alpha-tocopherol, or both as treatment for Alzheimer's disease. *N Engl J Med* 1997; 17: 1216–17.

42 American Psychiatric Association. Practice guideline for the treatment of patients with Alzheimer's disease and other dementias of late life. *Am J Psychiatry* 1997; 154 (5 Suppl.): 1–39.

43 Le Bars PL, Katz MM, Berman N *et al.* A placebo-controlled, double-blind, randomized trial of an extract of *Ginkgo biloba* for dementia. *JAMA* 1997; 278: 1327–32.

43a Anonymous. Dementia diagnosis and treatment. *Bandolier* 1998; 5 (2): 2–3.

44 Oken BS, Storzbach DM, Kaye JA. The efficacy of *Ginkgo biloba* on cognitive function in Alzheimer's disease. *Arch Neurol* 1998; 55: 1409–15.

45 McGeer PL, Schulzer M, McGeer EG. Arthritis and anti-inflammatory agents as possible protective factors for Alzheimer's disease: a review of 17 epidemiologic studies. *Neurology* 1996; 47: 425–32.

46 Stewart WF, Kawas C, Corrada M, Metter EJ. Risk of Alzheimer's disease and duration of NSAID use. *Neurology* 1997; 48: 626–32.

47 Rogers J, Kirby LC, Hempelman SR *et al.* Clinical trial of indomethacin in Alzheimer's disease. *Neurology* 1993; 43: 1609–11.

48 Aisen PS, Marin D, Altstiel L *et al.* A pilot study of prednisone in Alzheimer's disease. *Dementia* 1996; 7: 201–6.

49 Yaffe K, Sawaya G, Lieberburg I, Grady D. Estrogen therapy in post-menopausal women: effects on cognitive function and dementia. *JAMA* 1998; 279: 688–95.

50 Olin J, Schneider L, Novit A, Luczak S. Hydergine for dementia (Cochrane Review). In: *The Cochrane Library*, Issue 3. Oxford: Update Software, 1999.

51 Flicker L, Evans JG. Piracetam for dementia or cognitive impairment (Cochrane Review). In: *The Cochrane Library*, Issue 3. Oxford: Update Software, 1999.

52 Williams PS, Spector A, Orrell M, Rands G. Aspirin for vascular dementia (Cochrane Review). In: *The Cochrane Library*, Issue 3. Oxford: Update Software, 1999.

53 Dewan MJ, Gupta S. Towards a definite diagnosis of Alzheimer's disease (review). *Compr Psychiatry* 1992; 33: 282–90.

54 Lebert F, Pasquier F, Souliez L, Petit H. Tacrine efficacy in Lewy body dementia. *Int J Geriatr Psychiatry* 1998; 13: 516–19.

5 Treatment of behavioural and psychological aspects of dementia

Virtually all patients with dementia will experience problems with mood or behaviour at some time. These aspects are often described as 'non-cognitive', 'neuropsychiatric' or more recently as the 'behavioural and psychological signs and symptoms of dementia' (BPSSD, International Psychogeriatric Association Consensus, 1996). It is increasingly apparent that non-cognitive symptoms are almost more important than memory and cognitive decline in terms of the burden to caregivers and the socio-economic costs. Non-cognitive symptoms are the main cause of institutionalization and are a negative predictor of survival for the patient. In their management, these symptoms may require considerable medical and other input as well as the use of drug therapy.

It is difficult to get an exact breakdown of the frequency of particular problems because different reviews based on different carers and patients come up with different numbers. A review of eight studies in 1995 [1] gave the mean prevalence values for problem behaviours in dementia (Table 5.1).

Drugs that may be of value include antidepressants, anxiolytics, neuroleptics and hypnotics. Yet such drugs can produce problems of their own with impaired mental and motor performance. Interestingly, cholinomimetic drugs such as the acetylcholinesterase inhibitors appear to have useful and important beneficial effects on behaviour in addition to their effects on cognition.

All of these problems need careful assessment; drug therapy should be considered not as the first management option but as the last (with the exception of cholinesterase inhibitors).

Table 5.1 The mean prevalence values for problem behaviours in dementia

Behaviour	%
Verbal aggression/threats	54
Physical aggression/agitation	42
Sleep disturbances	38
Restlessness	38
Wandering	30
Apathy/withdrawal	27

Assessment of behavioural and psychological signs and symptoms of dementia

Careful assessment of any behavioural disorder such as agitation or aggression is vital in trying to determine the cause and the best way of managing it.

It is important to obtain a detailed description of the problem, its severity and frequency. Broad descriptions such as 'wanders', or 'aggression' are unhelpful and open to different interpretations. A person in a nursing home may 'wander' when their bladder is full and they cannot remember where the toilet is, they can 'wander' by trying to leave and go back to their own home, or they may 'wander' by continuously pacing up and down. Clearly these behaviours may have different underlying causes and equally should be managed in different ways. It is useful to note anything that triggers the behaviour (e.g. in response to a particular individual or a situation such as being helped to bathe); the behaviour itself (e.g. if the person tries to hit the member of staff when being helped into the bath); and who the behaviour troubles. Is it the person with dementia who is troubled or a family carer? In a residential setting is it the person, other residents or staff? If someone wanders undistressed around a nursing home without upsetting others, then specific management is unnecessary.

Management of difficult behaviour must be dealt with on an individual basis and the situation reviewed regularly. Unless the symptoms are extremely distressing, it is reasonable to monitor the disturbance for at least 1 month before starting pharmacological treatments [2]. This allows spontaneous resolution and the use of non-drug approaches.

Non-drug interventions

A recent National Clinical Guideline for use in Scotland has dealt with interventions in the management of behavioural and psychological aspects of dementia [3]. Quite correctly, this guideline emphasizes that on the basis of available evidence and the problems associated with drugs, non-drug interventions should always be considered before drug treatment is started.

Unfortunately it is difficult to assess non-drug interventions using rigorous methodology such as double-blind designs and placebo controls. Many are anecdotal and rely on individual enthusiasts; they do not necessarily translate successfully in a more generalized way. Where there are benefits they do not usually last longer than the duration of the intervention [4]. Although firm evidence is lacking, they may improve the quality of life for patients if for no other reason than giving them stimulation and increasing enthusiasm among staff and caregivers.

The interventions that have been described may differ in their focus, methods and underlying philosophy. However, they usually have similar goals to try and improve quality of life and to maximize residual function. In addition, they may be intended to improve cognitive function, behaviour or mood [4]. They are relatively non-specific in their actions and, apart from strategies to help with sleep disturbance, will be discussed together in the following few sections.

Behaviour-orientated approaches

Behavioural intervention involves modifying the triggers and consequences of a particular problem behaviour. The context in which the behaviour occurs is analysed in detail as are any regular antecedents that trigger the behaviour and the consequences of the behaviour itself.

Emotion-orientated approaches

These approaches include supportive psychotherapy, reminiscence therapy, validation therapy (which seeks to restore self-worth and decrease stress by validating emotional ties to the past), sensory integration, and simulated presence therapy (whereby simulating the presence of a familiar situation or person may reduce problem behaviours associated with social isolation).

Cognition-orientated approaches

These techniques include reality orientation and skills training. They aim to redress cognitive deficits often in a classroom setting. Reality orientation (RO) involves providing accurate information designed to orientate the person to his or her surroundings. Modest transient improvements in verbal orientation have been shown but there are also case reports of anger, frustration and depression precipitated by RO [5].

Stimulation-orientated approaches

These approaches include activities or recreational therapies such as games and art therapies such as music and dance. The goal is to increase the number of pleasant activities and this can improve the mood of patients and carers alike. Some of these stimulation treatments ought to be considered as standard in the provision of normal care.

Caregiver-based approaches

There is increasing interest in strategies that may enhance the quality of life of care providers as well as patients. Although well-controlled data are limited, preliminary studies and clinical practice support their effectiveness [6]. For example, caregiver-based behavioural treatment programmes appear to significantly reduce depression in patients for at least 6 months after the behaviour therapy [7] and also benefit the caregiver. The core of these programmes has focused on educational activities and stimulation-orientated approaches.

In long-term care facilities there may be benefits in training and education of staff. A recent randomized controlled trial gives preliminary support for this [8]. A programme of staff training and psychosocial management of elderly residents' behavioural problems in nursing and residential homes significantly improved depression and cognitive impairment; interestingly there was no apparent change in behaviour rating.

The role of cholinergic dysfunction in the behavioural changes of Alzheimer's disease and other dementias

There is increasing evidence that cholinergic dysfunction plays an important part not only in the intellectual deficits of dementia but also in the neuropsychiatric manifestations of Alzheimer's disease (AD) [9] and other dementias including dementia with Lewy bodies (DLB). Acetylcholine is synthesized in the basal forebrain in an area called the nucleus basalis of Meynert. The nucleus basalis is situated between limbic afferents and cortical efferents where it can potentially disrupt emotional function. Psychosis in DLB has been correlated with the cholinergic deficit. Delusions are common in AD, occurring in 50% or more of patients at some time or other, and may improve with cholinergic drug treatment such as physostigmine. On the other hand, anticholinergic drug toxicity is often manifested by delusions and these are also helped by physostigmine [9]. Other neuropsychiatric symptoms such as agitation, anxiety, disinhibition, purposeless motor behaviours and apathy have also been reported to improve with physostigmine treatment or with tacrine, sometimes independently of any cognitive response [10].

Encouraging information is emerging from the secondary analysis of trials with cholinesterase inhibitors suggesting that 50% or more of patients with psychotic symptoms experience improvement [2]. The results must be interpreted cautiously since patients were not recruited because of psychotic symptoms and placebo response rates are also high; more specific studies are clearly warranted.

Clinical experience with drugs like donepezil clearly indicates a noticeable reduction in the apathy that is a common feature of patients with AD. This may be especially helpful because apathy is frequently demoralizing to the carer and the literature concerning its effective treatment is sparse.

Finally, more recent clinical trials with the cholinesterase inhibitor metrifonate have demonstrated a significant improvement not only in cognitive function and global assessment but also in behaviour (see Chapter 4, p. 51) as assessed by the Neuropsychiatric Inventory (NPI). These are probably the first prospective double-blind studies to demonstrate that a cholinesterase inhibitor can show concurrent cognitive, global and behavioural benefit (although earlier studies with metrifonate and other drugs would not have included behavioural instruments like the NPI).

As a result, it has been suggested that cholinergic agents are unique psychotropic agents that will exert beneficial effects only in diseases like AD where there is a cholinergic deficit [11]. It is reasonable therefore to consider these drugs as first-line agents in managing behaviour such as apathy, psychosis, agitation and aberrant motor behaviour before considering other drug therapy, particularly if there would also be a benefit from any potential cognitive improvements.

Treatment of psychosis and agitation in dementia

Agitation is difficult to define and refers to a range of behavioural disturbances including verbal and physical aggression, shouting, hyperactivity and disinhibition. Psychotic symptoms include paranoia, delusions and hallucinations. Both these problems are common in dementias such as AD particularly in the middle and later stages of the illness. They are among the most common reasons for institutionalization and for specialist referral [6].

The problem must be assessed carefully to try to understand the behaviour and ensure that other conditions such as depression, pain, loss of sleep and unaddressed interpersonal or emotional issues are not overlooked [6].

Neuroleptic drugs are the main agents used. For many years there has been concern that these drugs are used inappropriately and too readily. In 1987, special regulations were used in the USA to control the use of neuroleptics in Medicaid-funded nursing homes. Although this led to the successful withdrawal of neuroleptics in 45% of patients, in one-third dose reduction failed. In 1997 a survey of people living in the community in England revealed that 51% of all repeat prescriptions for neuroleptics were for elderly people of whom 55% were living in nursing or residential homes.

Neuroleptics are targeted at psychotic symptoms including paranoia, delusions and hallucinations. However, agitation is possibly the commonest behaviour for which they are prescribed. The evidence for the efficacy of neuroleptic drugs from double-blind, placebo-controlled trials is limited. A meta-analysis published in 1990 [12] only found seven adequate trials. They did show a modest improvement in behavioural symptoms of inpatients with agitated dementia; 59% of those taking antipsychotics improved but so did 41% of those taking placebo, an 18% advantage of drug over placebo.

There are problems with the trial results because there is a lack of general consistency in patient selection, the nature of the dementia studied, and the definition of the behaviours being treated (which may have different neurochemical bases). The studies involved classical neuroleptics given mainly to inpatients. There appears to be little difference between thioridazine and haloperidol, with suspicion, hallucinations and agitation responding best.

There is increasing clinical evidence to suggest that the newer atypical antipsychotics such as risperidone, olanzapine, quetiapine and clozapine may be better [6]. Low doses appear to be effective, there is a reduced risk of extrapyramidal (EPS) and other side-effects, and they do not appear to have any adverse effects on cognition. Both risperidone and olanzapine have been evaluated in double-blind placebo-controlled trials in institutionalized patients with dementia. In a study involving 206 patients, olanzapine, 5 and 10 mg/day, significantly reduced agitation, aggression and psychosis without EPS [13]. In the risperidone study, 625 patients were randomized to receive either placebo, 0.5, 1 or 2 mg/day of the drug. Risperidone was most effective for psychosis and behavioural disturbances at 1 and 2 mg/day with no increase in EPS in comparison with placebo for 0.5 and 1 mg/day [14]. Risperidone has also been compared in a randomized trial with placebo and haloperidol [15]. Low-dose risperidone (mean 1.1 mg/day) was well tolerated with a severity of EPS that did not differ significantly from placebo but was less than that of haloperidol. There was a significantly greater reduction in the BEHAVE-AD aggressiveness score with risperidone than haloperiodol at week 12.

Other agents that sometimes appear to be helpful [4] include carbamazepine, valproate and lithium for acute agitation, rage and mood lability. In addition the 5-hydroxytryptophan modulator trazodone, β-adrenergic blockers (propranolol and pindolol), selegiline, benzodiazepines and buspirone have been used for agitation. There are few data from well-controlled trials for any of these interventions but they do seem to offer alternatives to antipsychotic drugs for some patients especially for those with conditions such as DLB where antipsychotics are not suitable.

When considering drug interventions, it is important to target particular symptoms and to set realistic goals for therapy as well as to review the situation regularly. For example, delusions and hallucinations in dementia do not continue forever. Doses of drugs used vary widely but low doses should be used initially, followed by a cautious increase where necessary. In general, lower doses appear to be adequate in dementia in comparison with non-demented psychotic patients.

Treatment of depression in dementia

Depression and related symptoms may be associated with dementia. However, the relationship may often be complex. Some patients primarily suffering from a depressive disorder undoubtedly demonstrate cognitive impairment that at its most severe causes a depressive pseudodementia (it should be noted that as many as one-half of people with pseudodementia develop dementia within 5 years [4]). Other patients with cognitive impairment, particularly if they retain good insight, will be depressed as a consequence, although at least one study has found no association between insight and depression.

In the past, depression in dementia was one of the few features that could be treated despite the risk of further cognitive impairment due to anticholinergic side-effects from antidepressants such as the tricyclics. Now, it is probably more reasonable to commence an acetylcholinesterase inhibitor and see what effect this has on the patient and his or her mood. An antidepressant may not be necessary especially if some of the observed 'depression' is related more to the apathy experienced by patients with AD, an apathy that not infrequently appears to improve with a cholinesterase inhibitor as discussed above.

Marked and persistent depression clearly merits medication. The choice of antidepressant should be based on the drug's profile and the patient's age and needs (Table 5.2). Since depression is often an underlying cause of irritability and agitation in demented patients, drugs with a sedating effect may be helpful. The reverse is required in apathetic patients.

Table 5.2 Choice of antidepressants in dementia

Tricyclics
Well-established efficacy
    versus anticholinergic effects (further memory impairment)
    versus orthostatic hypotension (risk of falls)
    versus cardiotoxicity (especially if ECG conduction problems)
Sedation: good (if anxious or agitated) or bad (if not)
Lofepramine, nortriptyline and desipramine less anticholinergic than
    amitriptyline or imipramine

Selective serotonin reuptake inhibitors
More options and fewer side-effects
    fluoxetine
    sertraline
    paroxetine (special care to withdraw slowly)
    citalopram

Others
    trazodone
    nefazodone

Whilst adequate dosing is important, most patients with dementia are elderly and therefore the minimum effective dose should be used. One side-effect worthy of note that may be overlooked in patients with dementia is hyponatraemia, possibly due to inappropriate secretion of antidiuretic hormone. It has been associated with all types of antidepressants and is commoner in elderly people. It can cause drowsiness, confusion and convulsions.

When antidepressants are withdrawn the dosage should be reduced gradually over about 4 weeks. Selective serotonin reuptake inhibitors (SSRIs), and in particular paroxetine, have been associated with a specific withdrawal syndrome.

Treatment of anxiety in dementia

Anxiety may occur in the presence of dementia and may be distressing as well as having an impact on cognitive and functional performance. It may also contribute to agitation. If anxiety is severe and persistent, anxiolytic treatment may be of value but it should only be prescribed on a short-term basis. In the past these drugs have often been used inappropriately, particularly in nursing homes and for too long without adequate review. This is no longer acceptable and has in fact been the subject of nursing home reform legislation by the US Congress.

Although benzodiazepines should be avoided whenever possible, they have been used to control abnormal behaviour. Randomized clinical trials, albeit often methodologically flawed, consistently show that they are more effective than placebo but not as good as antipsychotics [4]. Most of these trials have been of fewer than 8 weeks' duration and used substantial doses of long-acting agents; it is difficult to extrapolate these results to the lower doses and shorter-acting agents that are used today. Side-effects include confusion, falls (sometimes causing hip fracture), dependency and rebound anxiety on withdrawal.

Benzodiazepines such as lorazepam on an as-needed basis for infrequent episodes of agitation are also useful to sedate a patient with dementia to carry out a procedure such as a tooth extraction. They are also useful for patients in whom neuroleptics must be avoided, for example those with DLB or severe Parkinson's disease (PD).

Oxazepam and lorazepam may be preferable since they do not require oxidative metabolism in the liver and have no active metabolites; however, they do carry a greater risk of withdrawal problems if used for extended periods and the dose should be tapered.

Buspirone is a newer anxiolytic which is thought to act at specific serotonin (5-HT_{1A}) receptors. Response to treatment may take 2 weeks or more and it is expensive. There is some limited evidence of efficacy for treating agitation or anxiety in elderly patients with dementia but further trials are needed.

Treatment of sleep disturbance in dementia

Sleep disorder is common in dementia. Disturbance at night may include poor or interrupted sleep, wandering and nocturnal confusion. It can also be part of a more general disruption in normal diurnal rhythms. These problems can cause enormous distress to the patient and any co-residing family but also sometimes to neighbours and more remote members of the family who may, for example, be telephoned by the patient in the middle of the night. The goals of treatment are to increase patient comfort and to decrease the disruption to families, caregivers and any other people directly affected.

As ever, it is important to be clear about who is actually being treated. Is it the patients themselves or is the treatment designed to reduce the effect their behaviour has on other people? It may be in some circumstances that the disturbed sleep pattern can be ignored if they live in a setting where they can be supervised without undue problems for other people [4].

Although drugs have a definite place in the management of sleep-related problems, all other avenues should be explored first.

Sleep hygiene and non-drug approaches

Many carers will have already tried elements of good sleep hygiene but it is surprising how often it has not been properly considered. Regular sleep and waking times, limited daytime sleeping, avoidance of excess fluids in the evening, calming bedtime rituals (and the absence of a television in the bedroom), and adequate daytime physical and mental activities have been tried [4]. Caffeine-containing drinks and alcohol should be avoided in the evening, and drug therapy reviewed. The timing of diuretics should be adjusted so that the diuresis is finished by the early evening. Donepezil is recommended to be taken at night, presumably to minimize side-effects such as nausea. However, it can sometimes cause disturbed sleep and nightmares, and in some cases these have been improved by giving the drug in the morning.

There is some preliminary evidence that early-morning or evening bright-light therapy may improve sleep and behaviour. Other approaches such as the use of aromatherapy oils are being tried but there is little, if any, hard evidence for their efficacy. None the less carers may sometimes find such approaches helpful.

Other problems

The clinician must also consider other causes of sleep disturbance including obstructive sleep apnoea (usually associated with people that snore heavily), pain, depression and prostatic problems.

Drug treatment

Severe and persistent insomnia in the presence of dementia may require hypnotic treatment but this should be used cautiously and only short term. There are no specific studies assessing the efficacy of pharmacological treatment for sleep problems in dementia or that compare drug treatment with non-drug treatment. There are some data for mixed elderly populations [4].

Chloral hydrate was better than tryptophan and placebo but not as good as triazolam. Zolpidem 10 mg was effective and without the daytime problems of higher doses in elderly psychiatric inpatients,

50% of whom had dementia. Clinical experience supports the use of small doses of neuroleptics (e.g. haloperidol 0.5–1.0 mg). Experience with benzodiazepines is less favourable [4], although short-term use of short- to medium-acting agents at low to moderate doses (e.g. lorazepam 0.5–1.0 mg, oxazepam 7.5–15.0 mg) is sometimes helpful.

Other problems can usefully direct the choice of drugs for managing sleep disturbance. If there is depression, a sedating antidepressant such as trazodone or nortriptyline may be best, if anxious a benzodiazepine such as lorazepam may help whilst if an antipsychotic is needed small doses of thioridazine may be suitable. If other problems are not significant, then trazodone (25–100 mg), lorazepam (0.5–1.0 mg), oxazepam (7.5–15.0 mg), chloral hydrate (250–500 mg) or clomethiazole (5–10 mL or 1–2 capsules) may help. Over-the-counter preparations such as diphenhydramine often have anticholinergic properties and are best avoided.

References

1 Collenda CC. Agitation: a conceptual overview. In: Lawlor BA, ed *Behavioural Complications in Alzheimer's Disease*. Washington DC: APA Press, 1995: 3–17.

2 Ballard C, O'Brien J. Treating behavioural and psychological signs in Alzheimer's disease. *BMJ* 1999; 319: 138–9.

3 Scottish Intercollegiate Guidelines Network. *22 Interventions in the Management of Behavioural and Psychological Aspects of Dementia*. Edinburgh: SIGN, 1998.

4 American Psychiatric Association. Practice guideline for the treatment of patients with Alzheimer's disease and other dementias of late life. *Am J Psychiatry* 1997; 154 (5 Suppl.): 1–39.

5 Dietch JT, Hewett LJ, Jones S. Adverse effects of reality orientation. *J Am Geriatr Soc* 1989; 37: 974–6.

6 Small GW, Rabins PV, Barry P *et al.* Diagnosis and treatment of Alzheimer disease and related disorders: consensus statement of the American Association for Geriatric Psychiatry, the Alzheimer's Association, and the American Geriatrics Society. *JAMA* 1997; 278: 1363–71.

7 Teri L. Effects of caregiver training and behavioral strategies in Alzheimer's disease. In: Iqbal K, Swaab DF, Winblad B, Wisniewski HM, eds. *Alzheimer's Disease and Related Disorders*. Chichester: John Wiley & Sons Ltd, 1999: 809–16.

8 Proctor R, Burns A, Stratton Powell A *et al.* Behavioural management in nursing and residential homes: a randomised controlled trial. *Lancet* 1999; 354: 26–9.

9 Cummings JL, Kaufer D. Neuropsychiatric aspects of Alzheimer's disease: the cholinergic hypothesis revisited. *Neurology* 1996; 47: 876–83.

10 Kaufer D. Beyond the cholinergic hypothesis: the effect of metrifonate and other cholinesterase inhibitors on neuropsychiatric symptoms in Alzheimer's disease. *Dement Geriatr Cogn Disord* 1998; 9 (Suppl. 2): 8–14.

11 Cummings JL. Changes in neuropsychiatric symptoms as outcome measures in clinical trials with cholinergic therapies for Alzheimer's disease. *Alzheimer Dis Assoc Disord* 1997; 11 (Suppl. 4): S1–S9.

12 Schneider LS, Pollock VE, Lyness SA. A meta-analysis of controlled trials of neuroleptic treatment in dementia. *J Am Geriatr Soc* 1990; 38: 553–63.

13 Street J, Mitan S, Tamura R, *et al.* Olanzapine in the treatment of psychosis and behavioural disturbances associated with Alzheimer's disease. Abstract, *Third Congress of European Federation of Neurological Societies*, Seville, Spain, 1998.

14 Katz IR, Jeste DV, Mintzer JE, *et al.* Comparison of risperidone and placebo for psychosis and behavioral disturbances associated with dementia: a randomized, double-blind trial. *J Clin Psychiatry* 1999; 60: 107–15.

15 De Deyn PP, Rabheru K, Rasmussen A, *et al.* A randomized trial of risperidone, placebo, and haloperidol for behavioral symptoms of dementia. *Neurology* 1999; 53: 946–55.

6 Treatment of other medical problems in dementia

It is important not to assume that every physical or mental problem a person with dementia experiences is as a result of the dementing process. People with Alzheimer's disease (AD) and other dementias are usually elderly and are likely to suffer from other acute and chronic illnesses. Evidence suggests that elderly patients with dementia frequently have other therapeutically important medical diseases. For example, one study of 200 patients identified 248 other medical diagnoses in 124 patients, and 92 of the diagnoses were new [1].

Careful and skilled management of medical problems is important for a number of reasons. Firstly, any illness may increase the patient's confusion either temporarily or chronically. Secondly, drug treatment of other conditions may be partly (or occasionally completely) responsible for impaired cognition. Finally, these problems can have an adverse effect on the quality of life for patients and carers.

People with dementia need regular review because they may be less able to report their own symptoms; this is especially important if there has been an acute deterioration in their confusion or behaviour. It is also important to ensure that they and their carers are included in preventive health measures such as annual flu immunization.

This chapter will briefly review the commoner medical problems that may be encountered, with an emphasis on their practical relevance to the everyday management of patients with dementing disorders.

General health issues

Vision and hearing

Communication is extremely important and difficulties in seeing or hearing are common in older people. The first element of memory is registration of information and this will be impaired if, for example, the person has not heard what has been said.

When testing memory and cognitive function, this must also be taken into consideration. The person should be wearing his or her hearing aid or reading glasses before commencing. People with hearing problems will do better in one-to-one conversations in a quiet room than with several people in a noisy place.

An annual test of hearing and vision (including intraocular pressure) is important. However, these can be difficult to carry out if the patient cannot or will not cooperate fully.

Simple measures such as removing wax from the ear, providing new glasses or using brighter lighting can make a considerable difference to the patient and his or her family.

Nutrition, anorexia and weight loss

It is important to remember the vital link between good nutrition and general health and well-being; this is easily forgotten in someone with dementia, especially when they live alone. Weight loss has often been considered as an almost inevitable consequence of dementia. However, this need not always be the case (and some patients actually overeat and indulge in bingeing).

The patient must be given, and if necessary helped to eat, nutritious balanced meals, as well as having ready access to snacks and drinks. Undernutrition is common and may contribute not only to muscle and weight loss but also to conditions such as constipation and anaemia.

Eating well is difficult without reasonable teeth. Dental hygiene to prevent gum and tooth disease, and regular dental check-ups are important.

Foot problems

Foot disorders often cause discomfort and disability in older people and can be the reason someone stops walking. Regular attention by a chiropodist will minimize this risk. This is of particular relevance in patients with conditions such as diabetes who are already at a higher risk.

Urinary incontinence

Incontinence in dementia is not always due to dementia. Therefore it is vital to assess the nature and cause of the problem including if there is urgency and frequency. The urine must be examined even if obtaining a proper mid-stream urine sample is difficult. A urinary tract infection may lead to incontinence as may the use of diuretics. This is particularly likely when a patient with dementia is physically immobile or slow, or if they are in an unfamiliar place and uncertain where the toilet is. Leaving a nightlight on may help the patient find the toilet more readily, especially if they tend to get lost indoors.

If urinary tract infection and constipation have been excluded, developing a programme of regular toileting that matches the patient's own voiding pattern may help [2]. If not, the cautious use of drugs such as tolterodine and oxybutynin may be of value. It seems sensible to use the lowest doses possible in order to avoid their anticholinergic side-effects; these may be more of a problem where patients are already deficient in brain acetylcholine, for example in AD.

Faecal incontinence and constipation

Faecal incontinence is less common than urinary incontinence but more embarrassing and distressing to patients and carers. It may lead to institutionalization. In dementia it can arise when the normal reaction to the sensation of a full rectum is lost. It can also arise in response to diarrhoea from any cause (including as an adverse effect of cholinesterase inhibitors). The underlying cause should be treated if possible. Non-specific diarrhoea may respond to bulking agents and antidiarrhoeal drugs or, if necessary, regular enemas to cleanse the bowel.

The frequency of constipation increases with age. It can be exacerbated by opioids, iron supplements, diuretics or aluminium-containing antacids. Immobility, an inadequate diet and the lack of response to the urge to defecate may aggravate the situation in dementia. Severe constipation and faecal impaction can cause secondary diarrhoea and overflow faecal incontinence; it is also another cause of urinary incontinence. Although laxatives may be necessary, increasing fluid and fibre intake may correct matters.

Pain

A person with dementia may not be able to explain that they are in pain [3], yet this is likely to have a serious effect on their ability to carry on normally. Retention of urine, a fracture or other sources of pain may only be apparent because of increased confusion, agitation or other changes in behaviour. It is important to be aware of this when assessing a recent alteration in activity or behaviour.

Painful conditions are often underdetected and undertreated in people with dementia living in institutions. In nursing homes, they are less likely to be prescribed analgesics than cognitively intact residents. Older people with dementia must be encouraged to report their pain and these reports should be trusted.

The most obvious causes of pain must be excluded. If the diagnosis is not clear, then it is reasonable to treat the pain empirically and wait for it to settle or for other clues to the underlying cause to emerge.

Terminal care

Dementia sufferers and their carers need counselling and support throughout the illness. Similarly, just as for patients with predominantly physical conditions, when people with dementia reach the terminal phase of their illness they require effective palliative care.

There is evidence that these needs are not met [4]: patients in the last year of their life were seen less often than cancer patients and their carers rated the assistance they received from general practitioners less highly. Yet the patients dying from dementia had health-care needs and symptoms (confusion, incontinence, pain, low mood, constipation and loss of appetite) that were comparable. Greater attention must therefore be given to the needs of patients whose restricted cooperation requires extra skill and empathy from medical, nursing and other attending staff.

Specific conditions

A number of specific medical conditions are important and worthy of particular mention. They are already risk factors mainly for vascular dementia (VaD). They are common in elderly people and responsible for ill health even in the absence of dementia.

Diabetes mellitus

While good control of the blood sugar level may reduce the rate of intellectual decline, it is important to minimize the risk of hypoglycaemic episodes. These are likely to be poorly tolerated and may lead to further cognitive damage. Therefore it is usually wiser only to aim for moderately good blood sugar control.

Ideally, newly diagnosed non-insulin-dependent diabetics should be given at least 3 months' dietary restriction together with an increase in physical activity. This may be impractical for carers and elderly patients who also have dementia. Elderly people are prone to hypoglycaemia from long-acting sulphonylureas. Chlorpropamide and probably glibenclamide are best avoided and replaced by others such as gliclazide, glipizide and tolbutamide (that has to be given in divided doses so that compliance may be a problem). Insulin is best avoided if possible.

Hypertension

There is good evidence for the effectiveness of treating hypertension in older people yet often there is reluctance to do so. This can be a particular dilemma in elderly people with dementia. Since hypertension is usually asymptomatic, patients are more likely to develop symptoms as a result of the treatment. In any case, compliance may well be a problem.

The treatment for any patient must be individualized but it may be unreasonable to treat hypertension too aggressively in severely demented patients. On the other hand, successful blood pressure control can enhance cognitive performance at least in patients with multi-infarct dementia [5]. More significantly, antihypertensive treatment is associated with a lower incidence of dementia in elderly people with isolated systolic hypertension [6]. Nineteen cases of dementia might be prevented if 1000 hypertensive patients were treated with antihypertensive drugs for 5 years. Interestingly there was a reduction in the incidence of both VaD and AD.

At present, it is reasonable to treat hypertension conventionally in patients with dementia. In most cases, first-line therapy should be a low dose of a thiazide diuretic (e.g. bendrofluazide (bendroflumethiazide) 2.5 mg daily) to which a low dose of a β-blocker (e.g. atenolol 25 mg daily) should be added in the absence of contraindications. If patients cannot tolerate a β-blocker (and they occasionally cause confusion) or are diabetic, then an angiotensin-converting enzyme inhibitor is preferable. The situation regarding calcium-channel blockers is currently unclear. There are data supporting an association with a lower incidence of dementia [6] and data suggesting that they are more likely to be associated with cognitive decline [7].

Atrial fibrillation

Atrial fibrillation (AF) is a common and troublesome condition affecting 5% of the over 65s and 10% of those over 75 [8]. Guidelines on the management of permanent AF are clear in recommending the use of anticoagulant and antiplatelet drugs to reduce the risk of stroke.

Patients with AF have a fivefold increase in stroke risk (approximately 5% per year) when compared with a normal age-matched population. The risk of stroke is reduced by about two-thirds with warfarin but only by about one-fifth with aspirin. The patients at highest risk are those with a previous stroke, those over 75 and those with hypertension, coronary disease, diabetes, heart failure or left ventricular dysfunction [8]. This group may well include patients with dementia, particularly VaD. Warfarin is not used enough in older people with AF probably because elderly people are at most risk from the adverse effects of anticoagulation. This is especially likely to be a problem in dementia where compliance is a concern.

This condition illustrates how difficult it can be to use principles of evidence-based medicine in clinical practice with older patients; clearly, the clinician must take factors such as living alone and having dementia into account when deciding whether the benefits of anti-coagulation outweigh the risks. Often the correct clinical decision is to use the less effective but safer alternative of low-dose aspirin (75–300 mg/day) or sometimes other antiplatelet drugs.

Medication

Using drug therapy to manage other medical problems in dementia is undoubtedly a two-edged sword. Medications, judiciously prescribed, can be of enormous benefit; on the other hand, they are a frequent cause of iatrogenic problems, particularly by producing further revers-ible cognitive impairment. Two other relevant non-specific adverse effects are postural hypotension and falls.

Virtually any prescribed drug may cause confusion, but it is espe-cially likely with drugs that have anticholinergic properties. Drugs most commonly implicated are shown in Table 6.1. Particular care should be taken when prescribing these drugs to people with dementia. However, if a patient has become more confused within a short time of receiving any new drug then it must be considered as a possible cause. Some drugs may cause confusion at any time, for example diuretics by producing electrolyte disturbances that may be exacerbated if the patient develops diarrhoea.

Renal and hepatic reserves inevitably diminish with increasing age and most patients are elderly. Weight loss is also common. Standard doses of drugs that the patient may have been receiving for years may become too large and need reducing, yet this is easy to overlook.

A final comment concerns neuroleptic drugs. These drugs are commonly used to manage behavioural disturbances in people with dementia. Apart from the danger of giving them to patients with dementia with Lewy bodies (DLB) (see Chapter 4, p. 70), neuroleptics may hasten cognitive decline [9].

Table 6.1 Drugs causing acute confusion

Drugs with anticholinergic properties
Antihistamines (e.g. diphenhydramine)
Antispasmodics
Tricyclic antidepressants
Antipsychotics
Antiparkinsonian drugs
Oxybutynin

Other drugs
Benzodiazepines
Alcohol
Trazodone and other antidepressants
Narcotic analgesics
Lithium carbonate
Digoxin
Diuretics
Antihypertensives (? especially calcium-channel blockers)
Anticonvulsants
Cimetidine
Steroids
Indomethacin and other non-steroidals

Drug withdrawal
Alcohol
Benzodiazepines

References

1 Larson EB, Reifler BV, Sumi SM, Canfield CG, Chinn NM. Diagnostic tests in the evaluation of dementia: a prospective study of 200 elderly outpatients. *Arch Intern Med* 1986; 146: 1917–22.

2 Jirovec MM. Urine control in patients with chronic degenerative brain disease. In: Altman HJ, ed. *Alzheimer's Disease: Problems, Prospects and Perspectives.* New York: Plenum Press, 1986.

3 Cook AKR, Niven CA, Downs MG. Assessing the pain of people with cognitive impairment. *Int J Geriatr Psychiatry* 1999; 14: 421–5.

4 McCarthy M, Addington-Hall J, Altmann D. The experience of dying with dementia: a retrospective study. *Int J Geriatr Psychiatry* 1997; 12 (3): 404–9.

5 Meyer JS, Judd BW, Tawaklna T *et al.* Improved cognition after control of risk factors for multi-infarct dementia. *JAMA* 1986; 256: 2203–9.

6 Forette F, Seux M-L, Staessen JA *et al.* Prevention of dementia in randomised double-blind placebo-controlled Systolic Hypertension in Europe (Syst-Eur) trial. *Lancet* 1998; 352: 1347–51.

7 Dinsdale H. Searching for a link between calcium-channel blockers and cognitive function. *Can Med Assoc J* 1999; 161: 534–5.

8 Hampton JR. The management of atrial fibrillation in elderly patients. *Age Ageing* 1999; 28: 249–50.

9 McShane R, Keene J, Gedling K *et al.* Do neuroleptic drugs hasten cognitive decline in dementia? Prospective study with necropsy follow up. *BMJ* 1997; 314: 266–70.

7 General treatment considerations

The treatment of the dementias is multifaceted. It depends on the stage of the illness and must be focused on the needs of each patient and caregiver. Patients' needs and problems change with time, and regular review is vital. Formulating a care plan with the family which considers medical, social, financial and emotional aspects is also useful. It is worth re-emphasizing that drugs are only part of any treatment plan.

Effective drug treatment for dementia is in its infancy; it is wrong to expect miracles, or to consider antidementia drugs in the same light as if they were merely another non-steroidal or antihypertensive agent.

Use of treatment protocols and clinical guidelines

The acceptance of the new anticholinesterase therapies for Alzheimer's disease (AD) has been much greater outside of the UK. Tacrine was the first drug to be approved and was licensed in the USA in 1993. Over the following 2 years the drug was approved in many countries including Sweden and Australia, not known for the liberal licensing of new therapies. None the less, the drug was rejected by the UK authorities until 1997 when it was approved (but never marketed) shortly before donepezil was given a product licence.

It is difficult not to suspect that concern about costs led to the rejection of tacrine rather than its benefit–risk profile. This is further supported by the reaction of many to the approval of donepezil. Yet generally donepezil has received widespread acceptance and approval by countries including Australia and New Zealand where cost issues are part of the remit.

A number of so-called guidelines for using donepezil have been developed in the UK. Many appear to have been designed more to restrict the use of the drug rather than to encourage its appropriate use in those patients who might benefit [1].

When to start anticholinesterase therapy

All current antidementia drug therapy directed at improving intellectual function is approved for treating mild to moderate AD but this is not always easy to categorize. Determining disease severity is a clinical decision. It is often aided by the use of the Mini Mental State Examination (MMSE, see Chapter 3, p. 25) where patients with mild to moderate disease usually score between 10 and 24. Mild dementia is sometimes seen with scores above 24 particularly in people with a high premorbid intelligence (e.g. estimated by years of education, educational attainment or formally using a test like the National Adult Reading Test). The MMSE may be misleading in patients with marked language impairment who may score below 10 despite still having moderate impairment. In these patients there is often a discrepancy between their MMSE score and their everyday functioning at home where they may still be fairly independent.

There are more formal ways of classifying dementia, and this is what is used in clinical trials to give rise to regulatory approval for 'mild to moderate dementia'. The two main scales are the Clinical Dementia Rating Scale (CDR) and the Global Deterioration Scale (GDS) (see Chapter 3, p. 30). These are too complex and detailed for widespread clinical use except for places like memory clinics and for homogeneity within research studies.

Cholinesterase inhibitors should only be given to patients with mild to moderate dementia and benefits will not be seen in all patients (a provisional estimate is that about 40% of suitable patients will respond). Formal assessment of cognitive function using a test such as the MMSE is important for aiding in the diagnosis of dementia and in assessing the benefits of therapy; this can also be combined with drawing a clock face (see Chapter 3, p. 27).

It is still not clear how early in the disease process drug therapy should start. Ideally the earlier it is started the higher the level of functioning that is preserved. On the other hand, some would argue that only minimal benefit will be noticed until the patient has clear-cut functional impairment. This question may be resolved when the results of major studies with rivastigmine and donepezil are available in a few years' time. These studies will examine whether these drugs can delay a person in the prodromal phase of dementia (with mild cognitive impairment, MCI) from developing a formal diagnosis of dementia.

In general, the dose of cholinesterase inhibitors must be carefully titrated according to the manufacturer's instructions. This will minimize side-effects, which tend to be seen early after starting treatment or after increasing the dose. Often the side-effects will diminish after a few days so that the dose can be continued. Efficacy may be seen after a few weeks but this should be more carefully assessed at 3–4 months to decide whether the drug should be continued (see below). If the drug is continued then reassessment of efficacy should take place at 3–6-month intervals.

When to stop anticholinesterase treatment

Knowing when to stop therapy with cholinesterase inhibitors may be difficult. Some patients may fail to respond while others who are stable or deteriorating slowly may be benefiting from the drug. Equally, there may come a point in the patient's condition when further drug therapy is inappropriate and probably ineffective. In all of these cases it would be reasonable to consider at least a trial withdrawal of therapy.

Early discontinuation, usually within 3 months, is necessary if drug tolerability is poor, and sensible if there are compliance or other practical problems. However, before deciding a patient has not responded, it is important that the dose has been titrated to the maximum tolerated within the recommended dose range. Lack of efficacy should not be presumed until someone has been at their maximal dose for several weeks. There do not appear to have been any specific treatment protocols for tacrine where the maximum dose of 160 mg/day will not be reached for 3–4 months. As previously mentioned there are numerous guidelines concerning the use of donepezil in the UK [1] and these are also, more or less, applicable to rivastigmine.

A major problem with the guidelines results from the limited long-term outcome evidence available. Equally there are no formal drug-withdrawal studies except using the results from the washout period at the end of the double-blind, placebo-controlled clinical trials with donepezil. As mentioned in Chapter 4 (pp. 42–3) patients previously on drug were indistinguishable from those on placebo at the end of the washout period; no particular evidence has been suggested for a more dramatic withdrawal effect with severe deterioration. There have been occasional reports of patients on tacrine deteriorating markedly when the drug is suddenly withdrawn.

In the review of 15 UK guidelines [1], most suggest donepezil for 3 months before considering stopping the drug, and a few suggest 6 months; two do not mention a time whilst one states it should be considered 'regularly' [1]. For donepezil, where 5 mg is given for the first month before any increase to 10 mg, patients at 3 months will have had the highest recommended dose for 2 months and this should usually be adequate to assess efficacy. Three-month assessment for response prior to agreeing continuation of treatment has been reported to select a group who maintain their response [2]. For rivastigmine, with its longer titration phase, the patient will only have been at the highest dose (6 mg b.d.) for a maximum of 6 weeks. There is a suggestion [3] from an open-label study of 44 patients taking rivastigmine that some patients showed improvements later than 12 weeks based on MMSE scores and clinical impression; 3 months may therefore be too soon to make a decision on initial efficacy.

Most guidelines are vague when it comes to defining lack of response or a poor response. Some recommend drug discontinuation if the patient declines below their own baseline score. This is not sensible since it is expected that patients will continue to decline and they may still be benefiting from the drug when they pass their baseline.

The decision to continue the treatment and in particular to decide when there no longer appears to be significant benefit is usually left to a clinician's judgement, possibly guided by measures of cognition and function. It should also involve the patient, family and members of the multidisciplinary team [1].

Interestingly the issue of when to stop therapy with cognition-enhancing medications is barely touched on in detailed treatment guidelines from the USA [4,5]. This confirms the difficulty of this decision and the absence of clear evidence. One guideline [4] does discuss the lack of data to guide decisions about using or continuing the drugs in severely impaired patients. A medication-free trial is mentioned for assessing whether the drug is still providing benefit and this may be of use at other points during drug treatment.

Since the purpose of symptomatic treatment is to provide everyday benefits that potentially will maintain independence, it may be sensible to reconsider drug therapy when patients move to live in an institution such as a nursing home.

Our practice when withdrawing the drugs is to reduce the dose gradually (e.g. with donepezil from 10 mg to 5 mg for 1 month) to see whether the carer or patient notices anything untoward. In some patients, even those who have progressed to severe dementia, we have noticed obvious deterioration in general function and behaviour that has improved with drug reintroduction. On the other hand, we have seen occasional patients who have usually been on the cholinesterase inhibitor for over 1 year and have developed agitation, where drug withdrawal appears to have been followed by an improvement in the agitation.

Overview of drug treatment for dementia

Table 7.1 is an attempt to provide a more general overview of the use of drugs in the management of dementia, although it does not consider all of the behavioural problems considered in Chapter 5.

Table 7.1 Overview of drug treatment for dementia

• Assess the patient with a possible dementing disorder carefully including formal screening instrument (e.g. MMSE)
• If cognitive impairment
    consider other relevant conditions (e.g. hypertension); treat as appropriate and review
    consider depression; treat as appropriate and review
    consider laboratory investigations for secondary causes and CT scan; if abnormal treat appropriately and review
• Establish that the patient has dementia
• Establish the most likely type of dementia
• If vascular dementia, consider sources of emboli (e.g. carotid disease, AF)
    if AF, consider anticoagulation
    give low-dose aspirin (unless contraindicated)
• If dementia with Lewy bodies
    consider L-dopa for parkinsonian symptoms
    avoid selegiline
    do not use neuroleptics
• If Alzheimer's disease
    consider cholinesterase inhibitor such as donepezil 5 mg once daily or rivastigmine 1.5 mg b.d. Before commencing, choose specific target symptoms with patient and caregiver and measure MMSE. Titrate to maximum dose according to side-effects and benefits
    consider vitamin E (200–800 IU/day)
    consider selegiline or *Ginkgo biloba* if cholinesterase inhibitors unsuitable or ineffective
    consider oestrogen replacement therapy for female patients
    consider psychotropic drugs for behavioural symptoms where necessary and for those problems that have not responded to cholinesterase inhibitors

Ethical issues

Dementia and its treatment raises many ethical dilemmas since the sufferers are predominantly elderly and the condition affects memory, understanding, expression, judgement and behaviour. Patients are therefore vulnerable to physical, mental and financial abuse and it is also easy to overlook their individual rights. It is even easier to preferentially pay more attention to the rights and needs of the primary caregiver.

A number of issues of particular relevance to assessment, diagnosis and treatment will be considered in the following sections.

Informed consent

It is wrong to assume that a patient cannot understand relevant information about the assessment of their condition and its management or about involvement in research such as clinical trials. These issues may be difficult and any information must be tailored to how much the individual can comprehend.

It is important to try to obtain details about a patient's problem from someone who knows them well, usually a spouse or child but sometimes a friend or neighbour. This should be done only after the patient has given permission and this is not usually a problem.

If consent is sought for involvement in research it must almost always be on the basis of both verbal and written information. There must be adequate time for discussion including at a further visit if necessary. Consent is also often obtained from the carer, partly as confirmation of the patient's consent, and partly because their co-operation in the project will almost certainly be needed too. However, a carer cannot override a patient's view or give consent in his or her place except very rarely where they have legal guardianship for the patient.

Post-mortem consent and brain tissue donation

Confirmation of the patient's diagnosis can usually only be made by post-mortem examination of the brain. This is important information for research projects and a way of auditing our diagnostic and assessment procedures, particularly in atypical cases; it is also something that families are often eager to know.

It is preferable to discuss this at an appropriate time during the course of the illness and not only immediately after the death of the patient. Forms for brain tissue donation and details of 'brain banks' are available through national Alzheimer's Disease societies. Brain tissue from patients with dementia and from non-demented subjects for control purposes are needed.

If the subject is approached sensitively, permission for post mortems will be granted in the majority of cases. General practitioners are particularly important in this process since it is usually they that see the patient to confirm death.

Giving the diagnosis

Advances in the accuracy of diagnosing dementias such as AD, together with progress in genetics and possibilities of drug treatment, have stimulated much debate on whether patients should be told their diagnosis.

Patients are clearly entitled to be given information about their condition. As with informed consent, the information must be appropriate to the patient's ability to understand and will probably need to be repeated. Written information leaflets where available may also be helpful. There can be no hard-and-fast rule about what the patient is told and this should be judged on a case-by-case basis. Care must be taken where relatives insist a patient should not be told, for example, that they have AD. Research has shown that whilst 83% of carers say the patient should not be told the diagnosis, 71% themselves would want to know if they had AD [6].

Clearly there must be a balance between the carer's concerns and respect for the individual autonomy of the patient. It is likely that more patients will be told the specific diagnosis in the future. This will give them more autonomy and choice and allow them and their families an opportunity to consider treatment options as well as to plan for inevitable changes.

Treatment of behavioural problems

Most patients with dementia will develop behavioural problems during the course of their disease and these can cause considerable stress and difficulty to informal and professional caregivers alike. The temptation to resort to physical and pharmacological restraints is understandable. However, it is important to try to respect the patient's independence and right to be treated like other people. The overuse of neuroleptics is common and has been discussed in Chapter 5; in the USA, the use of these drugs in nursing homes has been restricted by legislation. The use of physical restraints is also to be deprecated.

Understanding the nature and causes of behavioural problems and teaching informal and professional carers a range of strategies will help to deal with these difficult issues and at the same time enhance the quality of life for patients.

Legal issues

The legal issues surrounding the competence of a patient with dementia or memory impairment can be complex. They will vary considerably from country to country according to local law. In the UK, the doctor is recommended to refer to an excellent report of the British Medical Association and the Law Society, entitled 'Assessment of

Mental Capacity: Guidance for Doctors and Lawyers' (BMA, December 1995, ISBN 0727909134).

References

1 Harvey RJ. A review and commentary on a sample of 15 UK guidelines for the drug treatment of Alzheimer's disease. *Int J Geriatr Psychiatry* 1999; 14: 249–56.

2 Evans M, Ellis A, Watson D, Chowdhury T. Sustained cognitive improvement following treatment of Alzheimer's disease with donepezil. *Int J Geriatr Psychiatry* 2000, 15: 50–3.

3 McMillan H. Delayed response to rivastigmine in Alzheimer's disease. *Prog Neurol Psychiatry* 1999; 3 (4): 28–30.

4 American Psychiatric Association. Practice guideline for the treatment of patients with Alzheimer's disease and other dementias of late life. *Am J Psychiatry* 1997; 154 (5 Suppl.): 1–39.

5 Small GW, Rabins PV, Barry P *et al.* Diagnosis and treatment of Alzheimer disease and related disorders: consensus statement of the American Association for Geriatric Psychiatry, the Alzheimer's Association, and the American Geriatrics Society. *JAMA* 1997; 278: 1363–71.

6 Maguire CP, Kirby M, Coen R *et al.* Family members' attitudes toward telling the patient with Alzheimer disease their diagnosis. *BMJ* 1996; 313: 529–30.

8 | Cost-effectiveness considerations

The costs of caring for patients with dementia are great and include direct, indirect and intangible elements. Direct costs may be medical or social. Medical costs include the costs for acute and chronic hospital care, physician time, medications and diagnostic tests. Social costs include long-term care, formal home-care support and environmental modification. Indirect costs cover the loss of productivity both of the patient and of the carer as well as unpaid services provided by friends or families; these costs probably form the major part of the overall costs but are often not adequately considered. Even more difficult to quantify are the intangible costs of pain, suffering and stress borne by patients with dementia and their families. It is difficult to measure the full and accurate economic cost of dementia yet this is important when trying to assess the cost-effectiveness of drug treatments.

In theory, the methodology for economic evaluation of the care and treatment for people with dementia should be similar to that used in other therapeutic areas. However, studies reporting the cost of dementia generate widely different estimates. This is because of uncertainties surrounding estimates of prevalence and incidence, the patterns of care and resource use, the efficacy of drug treatments, and the economic methodology and costs that are included.

The costs of dementia

General costs

The 1991 net cost of dementia in Canada has been estimated as at least $C3.9 billion [1], equivalent to 5.8% of the nation's total health-care costs. In the USA, the direct costs of Alzheimer's disease (AD) for the same year were estimated at $20.6 billion and the total cost $67.3 billion. The total cost (direct and indirect) per patient from diagnosis to death was about $174 000 assuming a survival rate of 4 years [2]. Much of the direct cost is covered by Medicare, Medicaid and private insurance, but families assume the largest part of the expense [3]. In 1991 Medicaid alone spent $5.7 billion caring for nursing home residents with AD. This compares with estimated total medical costs of $4.2 billion for AIDS in the USA [2].

The estimated cost of AD in the UK for 1996 is about £5500 million [4]. The NHS and local authorities pay 42% of this, the rest being borne by the Department of Social Security or by the patient and family. The overall cost is estimated to increase to around £7500 million by the year 2021.

Direct costs per year for patients in the community range between about $5000 in Canada [1] and $12 000 in the USA.

People with dementia living at home use a wide range of services. These include community medical, nursing and social support as well as respite care and sitting services. A recent UK study [5] has costed care in the community for non-institutionalized patients with probable AD. Costs associated with different severities of AD were compared with a matched control group over 3 months. The total mean cost per control subject (£387) was minor compared with the mean cost for patients with mild (£6616), moderate (£10 250) and severe (£13 593) AD. Indirect costs, mainly time spent by caregivers, may have been overestimated but were 68.6% of the costs while direct medical costs were very significant at 24.7%.

The costs of informal care

Most care within the community is provided informally and unpaid, usually by family and friends. People with dementia become increasingly dependent on others for help with daily living activities. In the early stages this support is mainly to help with more complex activities such as shopping and dealing with financial affairs. Later it includes even basic activities like dressing, bathing and going to the toilet. The situation often becomes complicated by problems such as incontinence together with all the various difficult and distressing behaviours that are part of the dementia syndrome.

The financial support provided by caring family and friends forms part of the indirect costs of dementia. More difficult to estimate are the intangible costs due to the stress and strain of caring after a loved one who is cognitively and behaviourally impaired.

Assessing the cost of this informal care is important when determining the overall costs. In a 12-month study of 187 patients with AD from northern California [6] patients in the community received as much as 70 h per week of unpaid informal care, mostly provided by one person. Even after institutionalization, there was a commitment of about 1 day per week; 31% of carers reduced their working hours and 30% retired early, with a mean time lost due to early retirement of 37–44 months. This may have a further cost in terms of reduced pension entitlement and can be serious for younger carers particularly when the patient is also young and with reduced opportunities for their own income and pension.

In the USA the cost borne by families caring for a person with dementia, including unpaid informal care and out-of-pocket expenses, was on average more than $18 000 per year in 1989. In the UK, 20% of carers aged over 80 were spending more than £300 a month on funding care [7] and 41% of carers had drawn on private savings and assets, taken out a loan or sold property in order to meet the cost of caring.

There are also hidden intangible costs of informal care. Carers suffer from a deterioration in health and increased health-care use [4]. There is an increased use of psychotropic drugs [4]. Most carers report some form of emotional difficulty such as stress (70%), tiredness (66%), depression (40%) and loneliness (36%) while over a third report physical problems such as back pain arising as a direct result of being a carer [7].

The cost of institutional care

Eventually patients often require residential or nursing home care. In many countries the cost of institutional care is the most expensive aspect of provision for dementia. In Canada the annual per patient costs of institutional care 'because of dementia' was estimated as $C19 100 [1] with figures of around $40 000 in the USA. In Israel the annual cost of institutionalization differs between private, public non-profit and government nursing homes and ranges between $21 000 and $28 000 [8]. Patients with dementia make up around 20–50% of the nursing home population.

The cost of drugs

In contrast, expenditure on drugs has been insignificant. In 1992/3 they were so little that they were not even reported by the UK NHS Executive [4]. This must be compared with spending on drugs during the same time period for hypertension and diabetes, chronic diseases that are less common than dementia, which amounted to 9.04% and 2.67%, respectively, of net NHS pharmaceutical expenditure.

In practice, the NHS bears a relatively small part of the cost of dementia at around 22–26% of the costs with only 1% of the total cost being accounted for by general practitioner related activities [4]. It is perhaps therefore not surprising at the reaction of Health Authorities and family practitioners in the UK to the arrival of drug therapies for

AD and their fear of the costs that would ensue in their budgetary sector. Most costs are currently borne by Social Security or, as elsewhere, by patients and families, many of whom suffer considerable financial hardship to meet the costs of caring.

Cost-effectiveness of drugs

Assessing the effectiveness of money spent on drug treatment with cholinesterase inhibitors and other new treatments is important. It will depend on the benefits from the drug and how these affect overall costs of managing the patient. If treatment reduces the need for support services or delays institutionalization by even a few weeks, it is likely to be cost-effective [4] to the public sector. Some allowance should also be made for any improvement in the quality of life for patients and carers; however, assigning any specific monetary value to this is not easy.

Acetylcholinesterase inhibitors

Tacrine

Tacrine was the first drug approved for treating mild to moderate AD. Results from a study using the highest doses of tacrine have been used to evaluate the impact of improvements obtained with the drug on expenditure for AD [9]. The net effect of tacrine, 80–160 mg/day, was estimated to save $2243 (1993 dollars) per year (range $-109 to $+3342) for every patient who started treatment, including treatment failures. Tacrine therapy could potentially have generated savings of up to 17% of the cost of AD at that time, or a total of $3.6 billion annually for the estimated 1.6 million people in the USA with mild to moderate AD.

Clearly, such estimates depend on assumptions made in the evaluation. The authors conducted sensitivity analyses for a range of assumptions and most demonstrated cost savings with tacrine therapy. Even the worst-case scenario only resulted in increased expenditure of $109 per year. In addition to the predicted savings, there are of course the potential benefits to many patients and their families through improved functioning and well-being, and a longer period of independence.

Previous economic evaluations of tacrine have also predicted reduced costs from institutional care. This is supported by data from one study [10] of patients who remained on doses greater than 80 mg/day in the longer term (minimum follow-up 2 years). They were less likely to have entered a nursing home than patients on lower doses (odds ratio > 2.7–2.8).

A more recent evaluation from the USA [11] has used the data from the above study [10]. Tacrine was associated with a per patient cost saving of $9250 (7.5%) from diagnosis to death, even when averaged over data from patients who discontinued the drug or took lower, less effective doses. Most of the savings were due to reduced time in nursing homes. The cost saving for patients who continued on higher doses was $36 500 over 5 years. These data were also robust over a wide range of sensitivity analysis variations. The authors concluded that, for mild to moderate AD, tacrine reduced the costs of medical and social services, increased functioning and delayed nursing home placement for up to 433 days [11].

Donepezil

Donepezil is undoubtedly an advance in the treatment of AD, and has been licensed in all major countries. In the UK its introduction has been difficult and controversial. There has been a failure to understand the potential benefits to some patients and their families and to appreciate that development of drugs for these conditions is still at an early stage in comparison with many other therapeutic areas. Some of this controversy appears more concerned with containing costs for a therapy that will almost exclusively be given to old people. Some highlights the uncertainty of many general practitioners in making the diagnosis of AD, or even dementia. Whilst the drug is simple to use, it has been recommended [12] that prescribing should be initiated and supervised by specialists with assessment of any benefit at 12 weeks. If general practitioners are to take over prescribing, it is suggested that this should only be done as part of a shared-care protocol.

After the marketing of donepezil in the UK, an early report of its potential value [13] concluded that the full economic costs of the drug could not currently be appraised and that there was no evidence to suggest savings to the NHS or any other party.

On the other hand, an evaluation of donepezil in Canada [14] predicts that, over 5 years of treatment, there will be a reduction in per patient health-care costs of $C929 balanced by increased caregiver time costs of $C48 leading to an overall saving of $C882 per patient. There is also a delay in progression to severe AD. These savings are increased if more AD patients are assumed to survive to 5 years but reduced if donepezil continues when the Mini Mental State Examination (MMSE) score falls below 10 (i.e. severe dementia).

A UK study has also looked at the predicted costs of using donepezil [15]. The analysis uses four sets of data: a cohort study as a basis to estimate rate of disease progression in untreated patients; the main

6-month randomized controlled trial of donepezil to give estimates of efficacy; mortality data; and costs of care packages for elderly people with varying degrees of dementia. A model was used to simulate the progression of patients. The use of donepezil was calculated to be approximately cost-neutral for patients with either mild or moderate dementia initially and therefore in favour of using the drug. Treated patients were again predicted to spend less time with severe AD where costs are highest.

Another study has used data from a longitudinal survey of carers of AD patients [16]. Patients who were not institutionalized at the start of the study and who received donepezil for 6 months were compared with those not receiving the drug. Mean 6-month direct medical expenses were similar for the two groups. The costs of donepezil were offset by a slower rate of institutionalization (5% for donepezil patients compared with 10% for controls).

A further paper [17] concludes that new drug developments for AD have the potential to offer cost savings for many patients and that cost-effectiveness improvements look probable. The authors also emphasize that cost should not be the only consideration in a humane society.

This paper also highlights one of the difficulties in considering cost savings in a country like the UK. Drug costs appear in the health budget whereas any savings are mainly in the totally separate social care budget. Such problems concerning inter-agency boundaries are not new either to psychiatry or to the care of elderly people [17].

Other drugs

Although there are few published pharmaco-economic data for rivastigmine or any other cholinesterase inhibitors apart from tacrine and donepezil, there is no reason to expect major differences. Tacrine is likely to be more expensive to monitor than other drugs because of its potential hepatotoxicity. The price of rivastigmine is generally similar to or slightly lower than donepezil, although the dose titration is more complex and requires more supervision in the first few months.

A study has already assessed the potential impact of introducing propentofylline in Sweden [18]. The study used data from a meta-analysis of four randomized controlled trials involving 1273 people. The costs until death were simulated for the 57 000 AD and vascular dementia (VaD) patients in Sweden theoretically appropriate to receive the drug. Costs of care were estimated from a prospective population-based study. The clinical effects of propentofylline translated into modest economic benefits even when quite conservative assumptions were used. The benefits would be even greater if a broader range of outcomes (such as quality of life for patients and carers and costs of informal care) were included.

Conclusions

There are now theoretical and actual data supporting the cost-effectiveness of several drug treatments for dementia with no hard evidence suggesting the reverse. A delay in the transition to long-term institutional care is clearly of benefit. It is now time to make these treatments more widely and equitably available. Future development of antidementia drug therapy must try to include economic evaluation within the clinical trial programme.

References

1 Ostbye T, Crosse E. Net economic costs of dementia in Canada. *Can Med Assoc J* 1994; 151: 1457–64.

2 Ernst RL, Hay JW. The US economic and social costs of Alzheimer's disease revisited. *Am J Public Health* 1994; 84: 1261–4.

3 Small GW, Rabins PV, Barry P *et al.* Diagnosis and treatment of Alzheimer disease and related disorders: consensus statement of the American Association for Geriatric Psychiatry, the Alzheimer's Association, and the American Geriatrics Society. *JAMA* 1997; 278: 1363–71.

4 Bosanquet N, May J, Johnson N. *Alzheimer's Disease in the United Kingdom: Burden of Disease and Future Care*, Health Policy Review Paper Number 12. London: Health Policy Unit, Imperial College School of Medicine, 1998.

5 Souetre E, Thwaites RMA, Yeardley HL. Economic impact of Alzheimer's disease in the United Kingdom: cost of care and disease severity for non-institutionalised patients with Alzheimer's disease. *Br J Psychiatry* 1999; 174: 51–5.

6 Max W, Webber P, Fox P. Alzheimer's disease: the unpaid burden of caring. *J Aging Health* 1995; 7 (2): 179–99.

7 Alzheimer's Disease Society. *Deprivation and Dementia*. London: Alzheimer's Disease Society, 1993.

8 Rothstein Z, Prohovnik I, Davidson M, Beeri MS, Noy S. The economic burden of Alzheimer's disease in Israel. *Isr J Med Sci* 1996; 32: 1120–3.

9 Lubeck DP, Mazonson PD, Bowe T. Potential effect of tacrine on expenditures for Alzheimer's disease. *Med Interface* 1994; October: 130–8.

10 Knopman D, Schneider L, Davis K *et al.* Long-term tacrine (Cognex) treatment: effects on nursing home placement and mortality. *Neurology* 1996; 47: 166–77.

11 Henke CJ, Burchmore MJ. The economic impact of tacrine in the treatment of Alzheimer's disease. *Clin Ther* 1997; 19: 330–45.

12 Standing Medical Advisory Committee. *The Use of Donepezil for Alzheimer's Disease*. London: NHS SMAC, 1998.

13 Stein K. *Donepezil in the treatment of mild to moderate senile dementia of the Alzheimer type (SDAT)*. DEC Report no. 69. Bristol: NHS Executive South and West, 1997.

14 O'Brien BJ, Goeree R, Hux M *et al.* Economic evaluation of donepezil for the treatment of Alzheimer's disease in Canada. *J Am Geriatr Soc* 1999; 47: 570–8.

15 Stewart A, Phillips R, Dempsey G. Pharmacotherapy for people with Alzheimer's disease: a Markov-cycle evaluation of five years' therapy using donepezil. *Int J Geriatr Psychiatry* 1998; 13: 445–53.

16 Small GW, Donohue JA, Brooks RL. An economic evaluation of donepezil in the treatment of Alzheimer's disease. *Clin Ther* 1998; 20 (4): 838–50.

17 Knapp M, Wilkinson D, Wigglesworth R. The economic consequences of Alzheimer's disease in the context of new drug developments. *Int J Geriatr Psychiatry* 1998; 13: 531–43.

18 Wimo A, Witthaus E, Rother M, Winblad B. Economic impact of introducing propentofylline for the treatment of dementia in Sweden. *Clin Ther* 1998; 20: 552–66.

9 The future

In comparison with many other medical conditions, we are still at a very early stage in our understanding of the nature of Alzheimer's disease (AD) and the other dementing syndromes. They represent a huge and increasing problem for society as a whole and more particularly for the individual patients, their families and friends. The disease requires a multidisciplinary team approach and it is right to emphasize that non-drug approaches are likely to remain a mainstay of the management of these conditions. Nevertheless, it is scientific and medical research that is likely to provide the most effective advances to help in our understanding, treatment and, eventually, cure of these conditions.

Advances in evaluation and assessment

Earlier diagnosis of dementia

As more effective treatments become available, it will be important to make the diagnosis of a dementia as early as possible. It is likely that biological markers, preferably in the urine or blood, or possibly more accurate imaging techniques will allow us to identify individuals in the prodromal stage of a dementing condition such as AD and therefore target drug therapies at these people. This will include people who are currently identified as having Mild Cognitive Impairment (MCI).

More meaningful assessment

There is a need for the development of a consensus on the most meaningful outcome measures when assessing the benefits of drug and non-drug therapy. This must include neuropsychological assessments, activities of daily living (ADL) assessments, assessments of behaviour and 'hard' end-points such as institutionalization and mortality [1]. Instruments to assess the quality of life of both the patient and the primary caregiver also need to be developed. Some of these will be of particular importance when trying to assess the efficacy of disease modifying therapies that may well have less immediate symptomatic effects. Proof of disease modification is difficult and will require long-term trials which are especially difficult, practically and ethically, in dementia.

Many of these issues are currently being addressed by the International Working Group on Harmonization of Dementia Drug Guidelines [2].

Behavioural and psychological signs and symptoms in dementia

More research is necessary to understand the background to these problems and their underlying neuropharmacological and neuroanatomical basis. Some symptoms may cluster together supporting a similar aetiology. For example, three clusters—overactivity, aggressive behaviour and psychosis—have been suggested [3] as may depression or diurnal rhythm disturbance as potential targets that might be related to specific brain biochemistry. Drug therapy, either existing already or developed especially, could then be used. However, such therapy needs careful evaluation with good-quality, randomized, controlled trials, as do non-drug approaches wherever feasible [1].

Optimal usage of current therapy

There is still a need to have more information about the current therapies, particularly the cholinesterase inhibitors. The dose–response curve for these drugs is not always well characterized and it is rarely possible to identify features that predict whether a person will be a responder or not. For several cholinesterase inhibitors including tacrine and donepezil there is a suggestion of a relationship between the efficacy and the degree of cholinesterase inhibition achieved in the red blood cell. If so, should patients be titrated using such a measure or until the maximum tolerated dose is reached (somewhat akin to the clinical trials with rivastigmine)?

If a patient fails to respond to one cholinesterase inhibitor, is it worthwhile trying them on another? For how long do the benefits continue and should the drug be withdrawn after a certain period and, if so, when? Finally, how do we demonstrate more clearly to funders and health authorities the cost–benefit of these therapies as demonstrated, for example, by delays in the need for services and support or by delayed institutionalization.

Novel approaches to therapy

As understanding of the processes that lead to conditions like AD increases, new opportunities for potential treatment become available. Unlike cholinesterase inhibitors currently available which are mainly, if not completely, symptomatic therapies, some of the newer approaches may modify or prevent the disease process. Two key features of AD are the neuritic plaque containing β-amyloid protein and the neurofibrillary tangle containing the abnormal hyperphosphorylated tau protein;

these are obvious targets for treatment. Opportunities for gene therapy are also likely to become available.

Anti-amyloid strategies

The key molecule in amyloid deposition is the 42-amino-acid form of the β-amyloid protein (Aβ) produced by abnormal cleavage of the amyloid precursor protein. Future treatment will aim to stop accumulation of Aβ or to remove it once it has been deposited. Approaches include the following.

• Inhibition or modulation of amyloid-forming enzymes such as secretases, for example through specific protease inhibitors. A cautionary note concerns the suggestion that such inhibitors (presenilin inhibitors) might be hazardous on related processes with negative effects on haematopoiesis and other aspects of growth and development.

• Decreasing aggregation of Aβ into fibrils, for example via anti-inflammatory drugs or antioxidants.

• Reducing the neuronal toxicity of amyloid, for example through anti-inflammatory medication.

• Immunization with Aβ. In a transgenic AD model in mice, this prevented development of plaques in young animals while reducing their extent and progression in older mice [4].

Anti-tau therapy

The presence of neurofibrillary tangles is an important feature of AD and several other dementias. Within the tangle is hyperphosphorylated tau protein. Preventing the hyperphosphorylation by increasing the activity of protein phosphatases might prevent tangle formation. Agents that modulate protein kinases or phosphatases could have therapeutic potential.

Gene therapy

In the future, gene therapy may well provide a solution to the problems of dementia. This may not be so far away with news in 1999 of planned trials in AD. Following diagnosis, skin fibroblasts will be isolated from patients and grown in the laboratory. They will then be transfected with a gene coding for nerve growth factor and the transfected cells surgically implanted into the brain.

Understanding more about those rare genetic abnormalities that are causative for dementias like AD and Huntington's disease may eventually lead to gene replacement therapy. Genetic factors such as apo-E4 increase susceptibility to dementia but are not causative on their own. Other susceptibility factors remain to be identified and these will give further insight into the underlying pathogenic process as well as offering therapeutic opportunities.

Availability of drugs for dementia

Concern has been expressed that patients with AD in Europe and across the Atlantic do not have equal access to antidementia drugs because of registration and reimbursement issues [5]. It seems unreasonable to withhold these drugs from patients with dementia on the basis of cost or because unrealistically high standards for proving efficacy are demanded. Of the three cholinesterase inhibitors currently available, they are fully reimbursed in some countries whereas in others they are either not available or reimbursed partially or not at all. In the UK the situation is even more inequitable since it depends on where you live whether the drug will be available and whether it will be prescribed on the NHS (so-called postcode prescribing).

It is increasingly clear that these drugs provide not only a tangible benefit to many patients and their families but also an economic benefit in terms of the amount of care that patients require [5]. Whilst there will inevitably be concerns by governments and regulators about the costs of drugs, this will be offset by even a relatively minor delay in institutionalization [5,6]. There must be a constructive dialogue between researchers, pharmaceutical companies, health and social service authorities, and the licensing authorities if patients and their families are not to suffer.

References

1 American Psychiatric Association. Practice guideline for the treatment of patients with Alzheimer's disease and other dementias of late life. *Am J Psychiatry* 1997; 154 (5 Suppl.): 1–39.

2 Whitehouse PJ. The International Working Group on Harmonization of Dementia Drug Guidelines: past, present and future. *Alzheimer Dis Assoc Disord* 1997; 11 (Suppl. 3): 2–5.

3 Hope T, Keene J. Behavioral problems in dementia and biochemistry: clinical aspects. *Neurodegeneration* 1996; 5: 399–406.

4 Schenk D, Barbour R, Dunn W *et al.* Immunization with amyloid-β attenuates Alzheimer-disease-like pathology in the PDAPP mouse. *Nature* 1999; 400: 173–7.

5 Winblad B. Harmonisation of availability of drugs for Alzheimer's disease. *Lancet* 1999; 354: 257.

6 Bosanquet N, May J, Johnson N. *Alzheimer's Disease in the United Kingdom: Burden of Disease and Future Care*, Health Policy Review Paper Number 12. London: Health Policy Unit, Imperial College School of Medicine, 1998.

Index

Please note:
All entries relate to dementia unless otherwise noted.
Entries have been kept to a minimum under both 'drugs' and 'dementia' and readers are advised to seek more specific entries.
Page numbers in **bold** refer to tables or boxes. Page numbers in *italics* refer to figures.
This index is in letter-by-letter order, whereby spaces and hyphens are ignored in the alphabetization process.